LOST IN THE DARKNESS
Lost in the Darkness
LOST IN THE DARKNESS
st in the Darkness

Lost in the Darkness

LOST IN THE DARKNESS

Life Inside The World's Most Haunted Prisons, Hospitals, & Asylums

Benjamin S. Jeffries

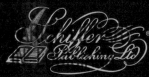

Schiffer Publishing Ltd

4880 Lower Valley Road • Atglen, PA 19310

Published by Schiffer Publishing, Ltd.
4880 Lower Valley Road
Atglen, PA 19310
Phone: (610) 593-1777; Fax: (610) 593-2002
E-mail: Info@schifferbooks.com

For the largest selection of fine reference books on
this and related subjects, please visit our website at
www.schifferbooks.com.
You may also write for a free catalog.

This book may be purchased from the publisher.
Please try your bookstore first.

We are always looking for people to write books on
new and related subjects. If you have an idea for a
book, please contact us at
proposals@schifferbooks.com.

**Schiffer Books are available at special discounts
for bulk purchases for sales promotions
or premiums. Special editions, including
personalized covers, corporate imprints, and
excerpts can be created in large quantities for
special needs. For more information, contact the
publisher.**

In Europe, Schiffer books are distributed by:
Bushwood Books
6 Marksbury Ave.
Kew Gardens
Surrey TW9 4JF England
Phone: 44 (0) 20 8392 8585
Fax: 44 (0) 20 8392 9876
E-mail: info@bushwoodbooks.co.uk
Website: www.bushwoodbooks.co.uk

Some photos are from flicker.com
using a creative commons license,
Public-Domain-Photos.com or
public-domain-pictures.net.

Text and images by author unless otherwise noted.

Library of Congress Control Number: 2013939945

Designed by RoS
Type set in vtks distress/NewBskvll BT

ISBN: 978-0-7643-4319-3
Printed in China

DEDICATION

To my amazing father, Arliss Jeffries,

who taught me to write from my gut

and live without regret.

And to my incredible wife, Diane,

who never let me settle for "good enough"

and loved me in spite of my interest

in the paranormal.

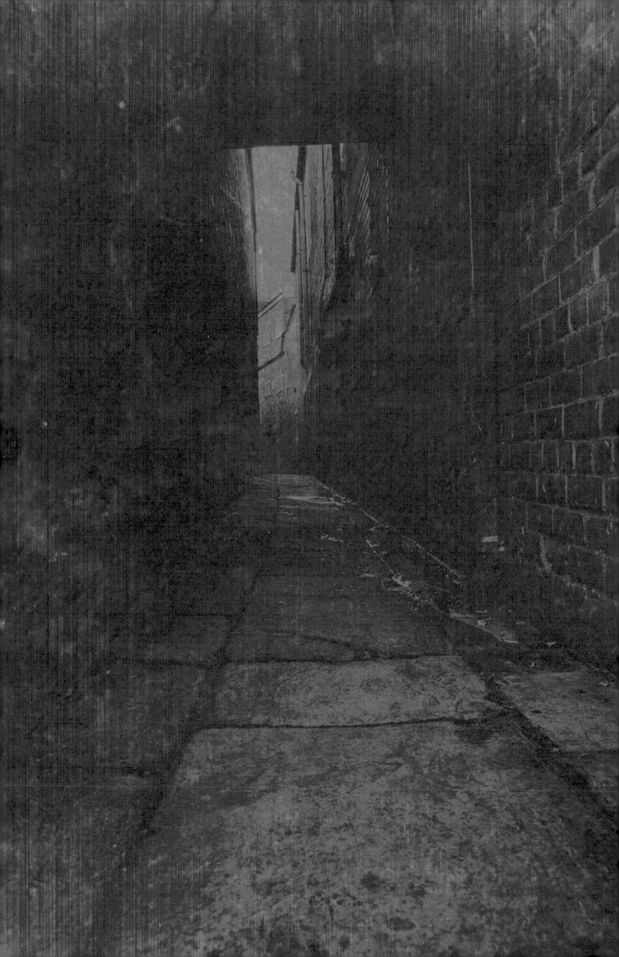

CONTENTS

PREFACE

When I was a kid, I was fascinated with ghosts and hauntings. It wasn't because I loved being scared; I didn't. I loved not knowing what was lurking in the dark. I loved that chill that would creep up my spine and nest there when I would pass a house in town that my friends had deemed "haunted." But while they crossed the street in order to avoid walking in front of it, I found myself wondering what secrets lay inside the old house, and, more importantly, *who* may have been watching me watching them.

A lot of people found me weird, a bit too strange perhaps, wrapped up in a world that both fascinates and repulses. I was a lover of the old-time campfire ghost stories and Arch Obler's *Lights Out,* which I discovered *a long time* after it had been on the radio.

It's been probably over thirty years since I was first photographed with a spirit lingering in the background of the shot, a ghost that haunted my boyhood home that I had named John.

Up until recently, there was a sort of taboo surrounding the paranormal. Some believed in it, others didn't, and still others thought that the only ghost that ever existed was the Holy Ghost. But whatever your belief, most people collectively viewed the paranormal as a dark, almost evil science when, in reality, it is more of an affirmation of the dogmatic Christian beliefs of life going on after death. I, in turn, was branded a complete weirdo, but I didn't care. This was what I liked; this was where I felt I belonged. I collected books, magazines, and movies about the most horrifying haunted houses in the world. It completely enthralled and fascinated me, but I never really knew why.

In May of 2012, I set out on a tour of the Midwest's most famous haunted locations: Central State Mental Institution, Waverly Hills Sanatorium, the Trans-Allegheny Lunatic Asylum, the West Virginia Penitentiary, and the Ohio State Reformatory. I had already written about them in the book you now hold and I decided that now was the right time to finally pay them a visit.

I had stopped at the Central State Mental Institution, which closed down in 1994. I was delighted in the fact that here was this grand old campus, rotting away in a downtown ghetto, and I was there photographing it and taking in the sight of what I had written about only a few months before. As I was walking around the outside of the Carpentry Building near the monstrous power house, I heard a voice, not four feet behind me, ask, "What are you doing here?" I turned, but no one was there. The fact that this was a genuinely disembodied voice didn't hit me until I had finished and had made my way off the property.

Then I realized...I really didn't have an answer for him. What *was* I doing there? What was my purpose in visiting the ruins of someone else's Hell? Was it to be a tourist and exploit the buildings and practices that may have created these hauntings? Or did I need to go to Central State and the other places in order to see them as they truly were, and not how the campfire gods and buff TV ghost hunters wanted me to see them?

The paranormal world is presented to us everyday in books, magazines, and especially, television shows. They're told as campfire stories and that's the extent of their usefulness in the everyday world. I saw it that way for a long time, too, but everything changed when I finally got to visit some of these places. Remnants of the past, such as diapers, old wheelchairs, and discarded utensils, were scattered across the floors. I found paper hearts made by patients for Valentine's Day still taped to the walls of Pennhurst State School, mirroring their inner longing for peace. The names of patients still linger on empty closets and cubbies in places like Waverly Hills. These too are ghosts from the past, written in time years ago by those suffering and begging for help in their own special way. When you see what was left behind, you quickly stop seeing the campfire tales and immediately begin to see the very real lives that were lived and lost in these horrendous monuments to suffering.

The stories of their hauntings are chilling and entertaining— I'll not deny that one bit. I relished telling those tales for you in every way. But the stories of their lives and the ways in which they lived reflect the practices of the times, which, by most accounts, were cruel, barbaric, and inhumane. These are practices and lives that cannot be forgotten, else we may live to repeat the horrors of past generations.

I saw neglected and damaged children being locked away and forgotten, beaten and abused by people they were supposed to trust. I saw hardened spirits, much like their human selves, still lashing out at a humanity that had shunned them from behind steel bars. I saw people haunted by insanity, left to wallow in their horror, instead of being treated and helped. I began to see the people hidden behind the moldering walls of prisons, hospitals, and asylums. That was when this book ceased being about haunted buildings and became a book about people—people still haunted by their lives, still lost in the darkness.

GLOSSARY OF TERMS

Orb

The most commonly seen phenomena in parapsychology. True orbs appear as translucent, perfectly round balls of light in varying colors, although white is the most common. Most investigators believe that orbs are the physical energy given off by ghosts and spirits. Orbs can appear on video, as well as photographs, moving in directions and at speeds uncommon for mere bugs or dust. True orbs are often marked by sudden drops in temperature and spikes in the electromagnetic field.

Anomaly

Any phenomena that seems out of place or character for the location in which it is witnessed. Twinkling lights where there are none is an example. The materialization and quick dissipation of mist or ectoplasm is another. The sound of splashing water in an empty swimming pool can be signs of both an anomaly and a Residual Haunting.

Apparition

The materialization of a spirit into a human form, so it can be seen by the living. It may be only a face or hand (partial apparition) or the full form of a human being (full-body apparition).

Clairvoyance

An acute perceptiveness that allows one to see things one cannot see with the naked eye. Also known as ESP (Extra-Sensory Perception).

Ectoplasm

The name of the mist that appears when a ghost or spirit materializes. Ranges from being thick and foam-like, to misty and smoky, like a cloud.

Electromagnetic Field (EMF)

A naturally occurring energy field that investigators believe is the main ingredient of spiritual energy. Can be detected with an Electromagnetic Field Detector (EMF Detector) or KII Meter, two highly prized tools amongst electricians and paranormal investigators alike.

Electronic Voice Phenomena (EVP)

The disembodied voices of spirits caught on tape or other recording equipment.

Intelligent Haunting

A type of haunting that shows some sort of intelligence through pertinent answers to questions or requests, or a curiosity and/or hostility the spirit might show toward investigators. Conscious or voluntary actions on the part of the spirit are considered examples as well.

Parapsychology

The science of anything that cannot be rationally explained or debunked. Literally means "beyond psychology."

Poltergeist

A destructive, fairly active spirit that tends to gravitate toward adolescents and teenagers. Poltergeist manifestations are typified by the movement of objects. True poltergeist phenomena is rare; most are elaborate hoaxes. Poltergeist hauntings can begin and end at any time, making their spectacle mysterious, random, and incredibly unpredictable.

Remote Viewing

A form of ESP used by psychics to become one with the spirits so that he/she may relive the experiences of a ghost or spirit in an attempt to reconcile the spirit's fate.

Residual Haunting

A type of haunting that seems to be a recording of a past event, one that may seem to play over and over again like a movie. Spirits in the midst of a Residual Haunting do not acknowledge the living and many investigators believe that it is not a haunting at all, but an imprint of some past trauma on the fabric of time replaying over and over again.

Shadow People

A type of spirit that appears to be made of black, misty ectoplasm in the obvious shape of a human. Psychics and investigators are split over the purpose of Shadow People. Paranormal investigators believe that Shadow People are just regular spirits trying to materialize, but lack the proper energy to appear fully human, thus creating a Shadow-like appearance instead. However, psychic mediums believe that Shadow People are spirits made up of dark psychic energy, can taunt, or lead the living to do bad things, or cause bad things to happen on their own.

Trigger Objects (aka Era Cues)

Objects or tools used by investigators to elicit a reaction from the prospective spirits during an investigation. An old teddy bear might garner a physical reaction from the ghost of a child, whereas a cigarette or snifter of brandy might entice a Victorian gentleman to speak. Music favored by the deceased may elicit a whirlwind of activity. The presence of an old Colt .45 might get the spirit of a gunfighter from the Old West to make himself known, and so on.

1.

THE WEST VIRGINIA
STATE PENITENTIARY

Moundsville, West Virginia

1876-1995

"I know what it's like to be ignored, and I think that is the big problem about the prison system: These people are being thrown away. There is no sense of rehabilitation. In some places, they are trying to do things. But, in most cases, it's a holding cell."

~Lee Tergesen
Actor, *OZ*

Deep within the caverns and hallways of the West Virginia State Penitentiary is a recreation room used by the prisoners called the "Sugar Shack." When the weather was bad in the prison yard, Rec Time took place there. It was a place to unwind, play cards, or perhaps read. A place where the stress of being incarcerated in one of the most violent prisons in existence can dissipate like smoke into the musky air.

However, in a place that was unusually unsupervised by correctional officers, it is but a major miracle that no inmates met their deaths in this now dank and decrepit room. It is a room that most certainly saw its share of violence, dished out by the hands of its subjects in the forms of rape, brutal beatings, and knifings with shivs. This is a prison that, at one time, ranked the highest on the United States Department of Justice's list of most brutal prisons in America, housing the worst of the worst of West Virginia's criminals.

Today, ghostly apparitions in the forms of an inky black "Shadow Man" appear on cameras wielded by tourists and ghost hunters alike. Disembodied voices echo throughout the cement wasteland. Attacks by unseen assailants, feelings of panic and distress, eerie footsteps, and the clanging of cell doors are commonplace. This is West Virginia State Penitentiary, one of the most active and thoroughly haunted prisons in all of the United States. And the Sugar Shack is only the beginning.

In 1865, ten acres of land near Grave Creek were purchased for $3,000, an attractive price for an attractive site: it was only twelve miles from the state's capitol at the time, Wheeling. But all was not well with the perfect location. According to legend, the prison buildings were to be built on old Adena Indian burial grounds. Indeed, the whole town of Moundsville received its name due to the large volume of Indian mounds dotting the landscape. Still, to this day, there is a huge, man-made mound behind the prison, housing the body of someone revered by the Adena Indians some 150 years before the birth of Christ.

Is the prison at Moundsville cursed? That is a question that can never be answered for certain, but the disturbance of a sacred final resting place definitely ensures a fair amount of unwanted and generally dark paranormal activity—even invites it.

As construction commenced, a temporary wooden structure was built, giving prison officials time to design and build the ideal penitentiary. In the end, they opted to mimic the style and architecture of Joliet's Northern Illinois Penitentiary. It was enormous, imposing, and inspired a large amount of dread in all who laid eyes upon it. A perfect physical and psychological prison. Ironically, it was the male prison inmates themselves who built the penitentiary at Moundsville, placing each sandstone brick into place as the monolithic structure became their tomb.

Finally completed in 1876, it boasted two different cell blocks, North and South, both measuring in at 300 feet by 52 feet. South Hall held 224 cells and North Hall held the kitchen, cafeteria, infirmary, and chapel. A tower that stood four stories connected the North and South Halls to the Administration Building, a wing that included substantial space for female convicts, as well as living quarters for the warden and his family. When the doors were opened and the facility began its run as home to the most brutal convicts in the Union, it boasted a population of 251 male inmates. When this phase of the building was completed, work began on prison workshops, such as a carpentry shop, paint shop, stone and brick yard, even a bakery and hospital.

In 1886, prison officials were exposed for using whips and other bizarre instruments of torture that were used to punish unruly and out-of-control inmates. A dismissed superintendent even explained the nature and inner workings of the "Kicking Jenny" (a full-bodied harness used to restrain prisoners for floggings) and the "Shoo Fly," a device that restrained the arms, legs, and head while a fire hose was unleashed in the prisoners face until partial strangulation occurred.

Still, despite the use of unlawful corporal punishment, at the turn of the 20th century, prison conditions still were relatively good, with education becoming a priority for most inmates with the construction of a library and school in 1900. However, this era of relative calm did not last long, as West Virginia State Penitentiary became known as one of the United States Department of Justice's most violent correctional facilities. How the tide turned against Moundsville is unknown, but what *is* known is that homicide rates at the prison began to escalate, and inmate-on-officer violence doubled. It can be argued that, as time passed, the inmate population grew and grew and grew, tripling quickly until three inmates shared a single 5 x 7 foot cell.

In 1929, due to severe overcrowding, West Virginia opted to double the size of the penitentiary. The 5 x 7 foot cells were too small to hold three prisoners at a time, but until the expansion, there was no other option. Two prisoners would sleep in the bunks with the third sleeping on a mattress on the floor. Once again, prison labor was used and construction was finished in 1959, delayed repeatedly by the steel shortage precipitated by World War II.

Charles Manson, famous for his role in orchestrating the "Helter Skelter" murders in Los Angeles, California, in the sixties, even wrote to the warden in 1983, requesting a transfer from his cell in California to Moundsville, purportedly because he wanted to be close to his old stomping grounds, he had kin-folk in nearby Wheeling, and because he "can't seem to git no mercy from Calif." His request was promptly denied with a very non-negotiable "when Hell freezes over." One can only imagine what life in one of America's most violent prisons would have been like had Charles Manson moved in.

As time passed and the West Virginia State Penitentiary continued to grow and nurture its reputation as one of the most violent prisons within the American prison system, a series of security problems began to lead to what would become one of the most infamous riots in recent memory. Up until that time, security had become severely lax, as convicts picked the locks on their cells and began to roam the halls without question or restraint. An onslaught of insects and substandard sewage lines caused the outbreak of numerous diseases that spread rapidly throughout the prison. Food was served with roaches and maggots cooked into it. Rats the size of house cats stalked the basements and kitchens. Now holding over 2,000 convicts, the West Virginia State Penitentiary once again faced the problem of severe overcrowding and worsening conditions within the prison.

But at 5:30 p.m. on January 1, 1986, twenty inmates stormed the mess hall and took six guards and a food service worker as hostages, binding them with their own handcuffs. They were beaten mercilessly and forced to take pills swiped from the infirmary. During the course of the riot and its ensuing violence, six inmates lay dead, slaughtered by other inmates, yet each hostage ended up surviving with only a few bruises and the horrific memory of that New Year's Day. Avengers biker gang leader Danny Lehman was chosen to present the list of demands, acting as the prisoners' ambassador. Of all of their demands, the only one that was agreed upon was the construction of a new cafeteria, one without dirt floors. Other demands that were rejected included the right to carry large amounts of cash and to have women with them in the prison.

Eventually, as the construction of more prisons began to increase, the inmate population declined to around 700 in 1995. But the fate of the Moundsville State Penitentiary was already sealed: in 1986, the West Virginia Supreme court had decreed that the 5 x 7 foot cells were cruel and unusual punishment. It took them nine years to decommission West Virginia Penitentiary and it finally closed in 1995.

But the damage had been done. Over the course of its 119-year history, the anger, horror, fear, and melancholy had taken its toll. In addition to the 94 state-sanctioned executions that happened there, an untold number of murders and suicides also occurred, possibly propelling that number into the thousands.

The late Paul Kirby, who served as West Virginia Penitentiary's deputy warden from 1992-1995 commented:

> This (prison) is not known for any reason other than being one of the most bloody institutions in the United States. My third day on the job, when I came in here, I cut a gentleman down who'd hung himself in our maximum security unit.

With only the worst of the worst populating the dank and cold halls, it is little wonder then, that West Virginia State Penitentiary's history of paranormal activity is so prolific, for when the lights were turned off for good, and the loud banter of cons and guards was silenced, the prison's real story began. Imprisoned in life, and imprisoned still beyond death, the West Virginia Penitentiary's spirits haunt their tomb like sentries, fiercely protective of what they believe is theirs, for if they arrived with nothing, then their prison is their only home.

In the words of Paul Kirby:

> If they die inside these walls, that's where their souls stay.

The Sugar Shack

The Sugar Shack, as mentioned earlier, is a small indoor recreation room, used only when inclement weather made using the North Yard impossible. Because of this, there were no Watchtower guards and rifles, and officers very rarely walked amongst the cons. This left the Sugar Shack open to fighting, gambling, and rape, to name only a few. Eventually, the rash of assaults and illicit activity prompted the Warden to shut down the Sugar Shack in 1979, its doors welded shut. It wasn't reopened again until 1998 when tours of the building began.

Almost immediately, experiences from tourists and guides alike began to filter back to the public, stories of apparitions of dark, mist-like figures, the presence of hushed voices, and an overwhelming feeling of dread and paranoia. The happy caricatures of people and animals painted on the walls only added to the spooky flavor.

As said prior, there are no records of murders ever being committed inside the Sugar Shack, but it remains a hotbed of activity nonetheless, most likely because this was the place the cons would have congregated while alive. It only stands to good reason that they would feel comfortable there in death as well. Multiple photos taken inside the Sugar Shack reveal numerous orbs, light anomalies, and even dark, mist-like figures, commonly called Shadow Men. Researchers have recorded unexplained bangings of cell doors, footsteps, muffled voices, and even the rattling of keys.

Apparitions of a Shadow Man, seen digging in the corners, have been witnessed by numerous employees, particularly at night. Why he is digging and who he is remains a mystery. He doesn't seem to care who watches him; the Shadow Man never acknowledges his audience in the Sugar Shack. This isn't the case for the rest of the building, however, as you'll find out. The Sugar Shack became a phenomenon of its own as reality television episodes of MTV's *FEAR*, *Ghost Adventures*, and *Ghost Lab* (to name only a few) staged ghost hunts that focused very heavily on this dark and downright spooky room. Their findings tended to lean more towards a Residual Haunting than an Intelligent Haunting, yet the evidence is compelling nonetheless.

The Ghost of R.D. Wall

The earliest sightings of ghosts at the West Virginia State Penitentiary occurred directly following the heinous murder of Robert Daniel Wall, inmate number 44670, in 1979. Known as a handy fellow on the outside, it was his job to tend to the boilers in the basement, making certain that they were kept lit and warm, maintaining them and keeping them in perfect working order. He had such a rapport with the administration that he was often allowed to remain in the boiler room—it soon became like a second home to him.

But to R.D. Wall, it may have been more of a haven than a convenient place to monitor the boilers. He was known throughout the prison for being a notorious snitch, a rat that couldn't be trusted. Being on such good terms with the warden and his staff didn't help matters, either. It never really mattered if he was a snitch or not; the fact that he dealt kindly with the Warden was enough to rouse suspicion in the other convicts and R.D. became a target.

On October 8, 1979, R.D. Wall was using the toilet in the boiler room when he was accosted by three inmates brandishing shivs, homemade knives that they used to stab and cut Wall to death. No suspects were ever pointed out and Wall's killers walked away from the murder. But almost immediately following the murder of R.D. Wall, guards and inmates alike reported strange sounds coming from the boiler room, such as voices, unexplained bangs and knockings, and even the shuffling sound of feet on the gritty cement floor. Outside the boiler room, guards watching over the North Yard would often see a shadowy figure walking slowly around the area leading into the basement, always between midnight and 4 a.m.

"I spent twenty some years over there on all three shifts," says former corrections officer Ed Littell. "Midnight shift; you're sitting up in one of the towers, you see shadows, you hear noises. You send a yard officer around to check it out and he doesn't see anything and thinks you're crazy."

Over time, they began to believe it was R.D. making sure that the boilers were still lit and warm. To this day, shadowy figures can be seen during the third shift, walking along the walls toward the boiler room. Even in death, R.D. is tied to his duties, a classic example of a Residual Haunting and a sad eternity to come.

The Murder of

William Red Snyder

In the fall of 1992, another legend was added to West Virginia Penitentiary's already storied past, that of the murder of inmate number 45512, William Andrew "Red" Snyder, one of the prisons most notorious and dangerous convicts. Interestingly enough, it is rumored that the character of Vern Schillinger on the HBO series *OZ* was based on Snyder.

A native of Weston, West Virginia, Snyder was an eighth-grade dropout and a member of the Aryan Brotherhood, a sect of Neo-Nazis bent on promoting white racial purity. Upon his arrival at the penitentiary, he spent a few years in the more mainstream wing of the prison, but was sent to the brutal North Hall in 1971 after he stabbed a fellow inmate.

North Hall housed the worst of the worst and they lived the bulk of their lives in seclusion from one another. For twenty-two hours a day, they languished in their cells, released only for one hour of yard exercise and one hour to take their daily showers. They ate together in a chain link cage surrounded by armed guards. The floors were made of dirt and the food smelled of rot. Life in North Hall was as brutal and unforgiving as you can imagine.

But to Red Snyder, it was home. To others, he was a cordial man when treated cordially, but like all sociopathic personalities, he could turn radically violent when disrespected or threatened. He was both feared and respected by convicts and guards alike. You would expect nothing less from a man convicted of murdering and dismembering his father and a neighbor in 1968, then stuffing the pieces of their bodies under his bed so that they could be "kept close." It was that reason alone why he was sentenced to life without the possibility of parole.

When the 1986 riot broke out in the main portions of the prison, many of the prisoners looked to fellow convict and Avengers leader Danny Lehman to help with negotiations. Lehman had been a model prisoner, was fairly well spoken, and had an incredible penchant for art; his paintings are still hanging up and can be viewed on the tours of the prison to this day. Quite the Renaissance man for being the leader of a notorious biker gang.

Being allied with The Avengers, Snyder found himself released from North Hall, where he began to take advantage of the random carnage that abounded. Six inmates were killed during that riot, but only one was attributed to Snyder. It seems that Red and inmate brothers Warren and Charles Franklin were the prime suspects in the murder of Kent Slie, a convicted child molester and murderer who was brutally killed during that same riot. Both Charles and Warren Franklin ended up being convicted for that murder, while Snyder's trial was declared a mistrial after a prospective witness was found dead, "stomped to death" in the Harrison County Jail.

The riot eventually came to a peaceful end and all of the hostages were released. Red Snyder went back to spending his time in cell 20 of North Hall. He was one of the old-timers, one who'd been around the block a few times, one who was respected as much for his candor as his menace. It is possible that Red's stature in the prison was the reason a man sitting in the cell four doors down began to fashion a shiv of his own, and it had Red Snyder's name on it.

Still, others believe that Snyder received his death sentence because he may have ordered a hit on Danny Lehman, the mouthpiece and face-man of the 1986 riot that got them a new cafeteria and sweeping new reforms. It has been stated in court documents that Lehman was killed by members of the Aryan Brotherhood, but Snyder's name was never mentioned in any indictments or testimonies.

On November 16, 1992, as guards were releasing convicts for their one hour of recreation time, Russell "Rusty" Lasseter exploded from his cell, pushed his way past the guards, and roared into Red Snyder's open cell. By the time guards had brandished their pistols and ordered Lasseter to surrender, Red Snyder had been stabbed thirty-seven times. Lasseter gave up willingly, dropping the shiv and raising his arms in the air. But the damage had been done. Snyder was dead and Lasseter's reputation was cemented forever. They say the attack was so violent that Snyder choked to death on his own blood before the severity of his wounds could take his life.

Because he was a member of the Aryan Brotherhood, it is a bit of a mystery as to why his death went unavenged given their propensity for violent retribution. Perhaps it was retribution from The Avengers gang for the murder of their leader? Or maybe Snyder was a loose end that was starting to come unraveled, one that needed to be cut off before it gave everything away? Perhaps. Whatever the case may be for Lasseter's motivation, it only got him transferred out of the prison at Moundsville. He was paroled a few years later, sometime in 2008.

Snyder's death was received as sad news amongst the inmates. Although he was a member of the despicable Aryan Brotherhood, he was so respected that the inmates took up a collection to buy Red a burial plot outside of the prison's pauper cemetery in the prestigious Riverview Cemetery. Though his body was received at Riverview, he was buried amongst the millionaires, socialites, and local politicians without a headstone, simply because he was a convicted murderer.

Murder happens regularly in prisons across the world, so what happened to Red Snyder should not be regarded as something special or out of the ordinary. But it is, for when Rusty Lasseter shanked Red to death, he unleashed a specter upon the West Virginia State Penitentiary that still stalks the halls today.

As visitors and paranormal investigators pass by Red's cell, they sometimes will catch sight of a dark shade behind the bars. Other times, the voice of the dead convict can be heard as clearly as anyone else's voice. His voice is said to be gruff, yet tinged with a weary sadness that is almost heartbreaking. Several orbs have also been photographed outside of Red's cell, leading most investigators to conclude that, years after his death, Red Snyder still serves his time behind bars. His voice has been captured on digital voice recorders answering intelligently to questions asked of him. When Rusty Lasseter was paroled, investigator Polly Gear and former guard-turned-tour guide Maggie Grey went to break the news to Red Snyder's ghost. As soon as he was told that Rusty was out of jail, they captured a weary voice on her digital voice recorder.

"I... already... know," it said.

The Shadow Man

While there have been a relatively short list of viable photographs taken at the prison in Moundsville, there is one that has become iconic: the infamous Shadow Man.

Rumors of a Shadow Man have persisted since the death of R.D. Wall and reported sightings have not diminished in the slightest. Yet photographic evidence has often resulted in only the appearance of orbs or organic, free-flowing mists.

That was before May 7, 2004. At 1:30 a.m., Polly Gear, a paranormal investigator with Mountaineer Ghosts Paranormal in Clarksburg, West Virginia, was alone in the North Hallway when she heard a noise coming from the cafeteria behind her. She walked back to the doorway and turned on the flash light to see what the noise could have been. Upon reaching the doorway to the cafeteria, she saw a black humanoid shadow walking toward her, staring out the windows to its right as it walked.

The light from her flashlight shined through this Shadow Man at the area near its arm, which caught its attention. It looked at its arm, then to Polly, and darted behind the door frame of an adjunct hallway. Fearing the shade would be scared off by her presence, she began to slowly back away.

The Shadow Man did not dart away. Rather, it seemed curious. Polly held out her camera blindly and took one photo. It was dark in the hallway and she was afraid that she had missed the doorway and the Shadow Man completely. But his image showed up perfectly in the extreme left hand side of the photo, narrowly caught.

She maintains that she was not afraid of this Shadow Man, indicating that a negative energy was not attached to it in any way. Had there been a drop in temperature, headaches, or feelings of dread, Polly's first instinct may have been to turn and run—not to pick up her camera. She felt as many of us paranormal investigators might: curious about the other side, just as the other side would be curious of us.

It is fairly easy to dismiss Polly Gear's claim that she photographed her own shadow or that of someone else's by mistake, or, worse yet, on purpose. But dismissing it vocally is one thing; *proving* it wrong is wholly another.

SyFy Channel's *Ghost Hunters* attempted to dismiss the Shadow Man photograph, debunking it by using highly advanced infrared cameras, infrared lights, and a flashlight. By using the infrared lights behind you, and holding an infrared camera, one could possibly reproduce the Shadow Man effect to startling clarity.

However, the Shadow Man in Polly Gear's photo is quite obviously the silhouette of a large man, tall in stature. It is obvious the flash went off, which would have drowned out the infrared lighting. If it had been her shadow, it would have been visible on the floor leading up to the door, which it is not. Further, Ms. Gear, a woman, is rather short with a medium build. If it were a direct reflection of light against the door, Ms. Gear would have to have been well over six feet tall and muscular with short hair. Ms. Gear, with all due respect, is none of those things. She maintains that during the private investigation, there were only fifteen people present, and only two of them were men. Neither of the two men were tall and as muscular as the shadow is purported to be. It is patently obvious that the photograph was not taken with an infrared camera, as the full-color spectrum of Polly Gear's digital photo differs greatly from the typically washed-out look of a picture taken with an infrared camera.

I have been to the prison in Moundsville and stood in the same spot where Polly Gear stood and shot my own version of her now-famous photograph. To fake the photo is possible, but not in a real-time kind of way. To stand where she stood and cast your own or anyone else's shadow would be impossible without it showing up on the floor leading up to the door; and even then, it would not be as dark, deep, or intensely black as it is. Then you have the option of manipulating it digitally. There are no tell-tale signs of any kind of computerized hoaxing involved, including severely defined edges, off-kilter placement, or the differing ranges of pixels of the image of the shadow versus the entire background. The Shadow Man looks and seems to be part of the original photograph and little to no deviation could be found.

What do *you* believe?

Incidentally, the Shadow Man would reappear four years later when he was photographed in the Sugar Shack by Pamela Tackett, a nationally known talk show host for the paranormal radio show *Coast To Coast AM*, who participated in an investigation in November of 2008. She was not alone, unlike Polly Gear, and her story is backed up by witnesses who were present at the investigation, seemingly solidifying Polly Gear's claim that the Shadow Man was real.

The Pentagram

In a wall in one of the towers overlooking the warden's quarters, renovators recently uncovered the astonishing stained glass sculpture of an inverted pentagram built directly into the window. It was only discovered when workers peeled away part of the coverings encasing the window. Sometime during its life as a prison, the window had been closed off, covered by cardboard and painted over to look like a solid wall. When the pentagram was revealed at last, it brought into question nearly every paranormal experience ever recorded at Moundsville. Had the builders intended the pentagram to be demonic? Or was it merely the off-handed use of a Masonic symbol?

Most investigators are split on these ideas, with many noting that the pentagram, also known as the Eastern Star in Masonic symbology, is inverted and circled, resembling the classic Satanic pentagram. Masonic leaders and scholars all tend to believe that, because the prison was made by bricklaying Masons, that the pentagram is merely a symbol of their presence at the prison, much like an artist's signature on a painting. It is inverted and circled not because of any dire Satanic influences, but because, as a stained glass window, the star would need to be supported in the frame better.

So, who do you believe? It would seem a bit overly dramatic to believe that the prison was built by Satanists to pursue their own evil ways and use the prison to collect souls for their Dark Lord. But if it wasn't meant to be anything bad, why was it covered up and forgotten? Perhaps because people got the wrong impression of it; maybe the window became dangerous, or it could be because the proprietors didn't care for it. One cannot easily forget the onslaught of demonic cults in the mid to late '80s when Satanic cults were supposedly in the midst of a renaissance, corrupting youths of America and defiling churches everywhere. Perhaps the hiding of the pentagram was a response to that.

Whatever the case may be, the once-hidden pentagram has now become a hot button issue that investigators and skeptics alike will continue to debate about in the years to come. Unfortunately, the original plans for the building have been lost, so we'll never know for sure if the pentagram was in the original plans or was added on later.

The North Wagon Gate

The North Wagon Gate is known for two things: how a prisoner arrives, and how he leaves. It is, for all intent and purposes, the alpha and the omega of Moundsville Prison. It was the very first incarnation of West Virginia Penitentiary, a two-story strong house that initially housed six convicts. Prisoners entered Moundsville Prison through this gate, and looking up, one can see how some of the prisoners left the prison, for the North Wagon Gate also housed the prison gallows. As the prison expanded, the Wagon Gate house was abandoned to the gallows exclusively.

Ninety-four men faced their deaths in this small building, their bodies dropping through the platform just above a waiting carriage. A simple slash of a knife and the body would fall into the carriage to be carried away to the neighboring prison cemetery a few miles away. To this day, investigators and visitors claim to hear the "clank-bang" of the platform giving way, though upon inspection, it is found to be unmoved and undisturbed. Occasionally, the slight murmuring of whispers can be heard coming from the room above as well, presumably a Residual Haunting of a past execution.

Psychic Impressions

Nancy Myers, an acclaimed Medium who has aided police agencies with great success in the past, has confessed that she felt very little energy in Moundsville's most famous building. But when she reached one of the upper ranges of the cell blocks, she was met by the tall, burly spirit of a former prisoner. The spirit advised her, in no uncertain terms, that she was not welcome on his range, or "tier." When she asked him what he did to get into prison, he responded with simple, yet chilling resolve: "Lady, I kill people and I enjoy it." Another spirit Nancy encountered seemed very well-groomed, even in his prisoner's uniform. He was adamant that he had been framed, yet Nancy sensed that he had worked for the Mob at one time laundering money. Research has indicated that a fairly large number of mobsters did time at West Virginia State Penitentiary, so the identity of this particular spirit may remain unknown unless he introduces himself.

In my own meditations on the prison in Moundsville, I came across the spirit of a large, frizzy-haired black man who referred to himself as "Caldwell," possibly convicted in the 1920s of murder. Though he did not commit the crime, he had a large hand in it and took all of the heat. He wanted to get across to me that he did it willingly without saying who it was. It seemed to me that he was protecting this person, whom I believe may have been a woman. An imposing spirit, but ultimately harmless.

When I tried to contact the spirit of William "Red" Snyder, I was met with a laugh as he used all of his energy to keep me at arms length, like he wasn't going to tolerate a long distance phone call, so to speak. He told me with that same chuckle, "If you wanna talk to me, you're gonna have to come and see me, boy. Ain't that easy."

In May of 2012, I had made my way to the prison in West Virginia, touring the place a week after they had staged a mock riot for the benefit of training law enforcement officers. If anything was going to trigger and rile up the spirits, it would have been that mock riot. As I stood in Red's old cell, I said, "Here I am, Red. I made it. Have anything to say?"

Nothing. The voices in the prison were eerily silent that day. It wasn't just Red; it was everyone. That cold, rainy Sunday, the Penitentiary felt like just an empty building. The spirits were there, believe me, but they didn't feel like playing with the tourists. A few times I thought I had caught something out of the corner of my eye, and I could definitely feel that they were around. But they didn't want anything to do with me or the group I was in. Not afraid; we just weren't worth the time. In Cell 20, I could sense that Red looked on me with a smug little grin, perhaps shaking his head in disbelief that I'd actually shown up. The best way to describe it, I suppose, is that it feels as if he had the last laugh. I came all that way to hear what he had to say, and he responded by shutting his mouth and grinning at me. Still, that's what I would have expected from him. I would have been disappointed if he *had* spoken to me. Well, not really, but you get my drift.

West Virginia State Penitentiary teems with residual pain that some believe is deserved and others believe is cruel and unusual. Whatever your belief, there is little doubt that the spirits are plentiful within the cold stone walls of a violent prison that has now become their sepulcher.

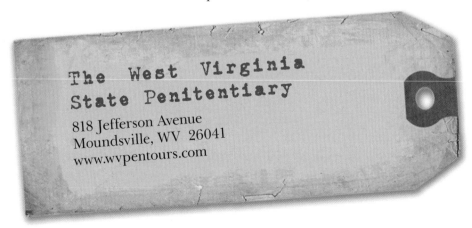

The West Virginia
State Penitentiary
818 Jefferson Avenue
Moundsville, WV 26041
www.wvpentours.com

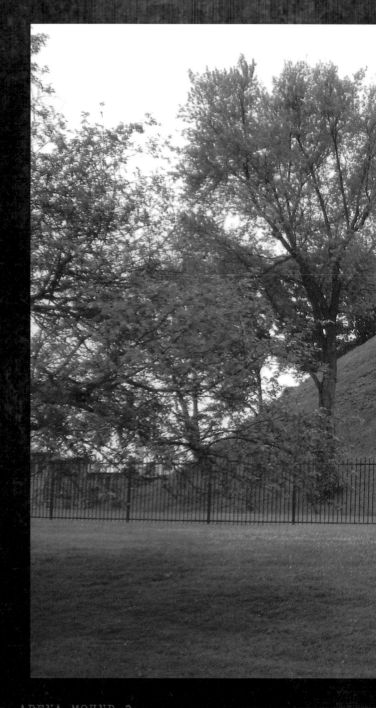

The mound at Grave Creek, right across the street from the penitentiary at Moundsville.

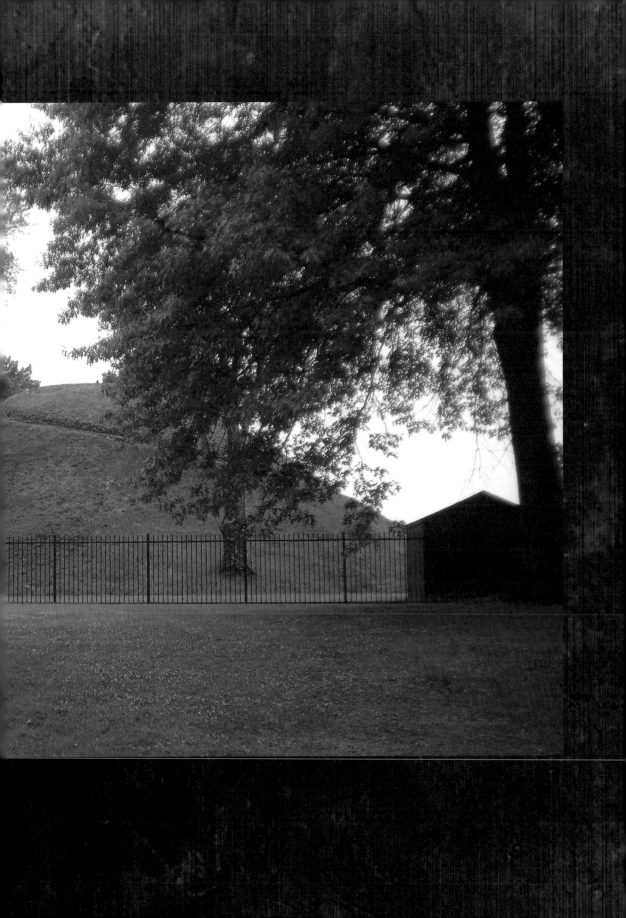

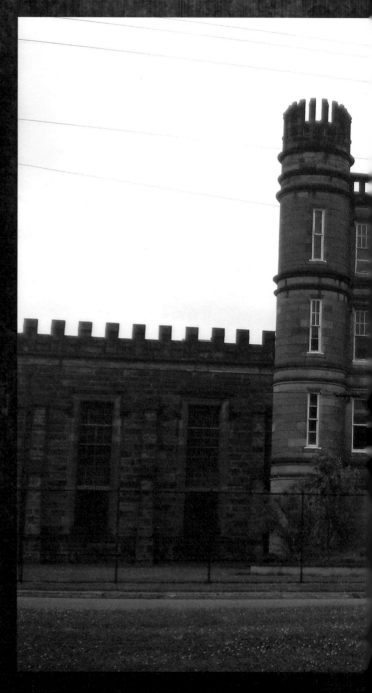

West Virginia Penitentiary in Moundsville, WV. *Photo courtesy of the author.*

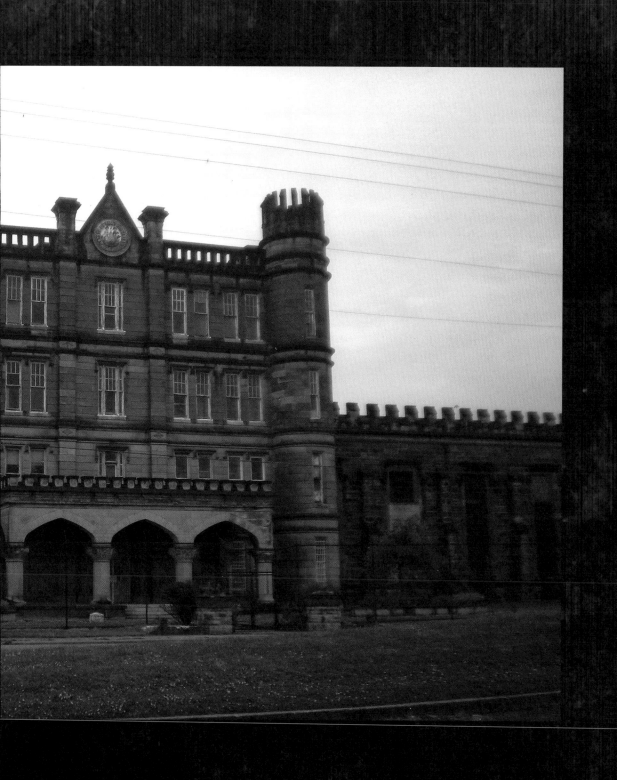

23

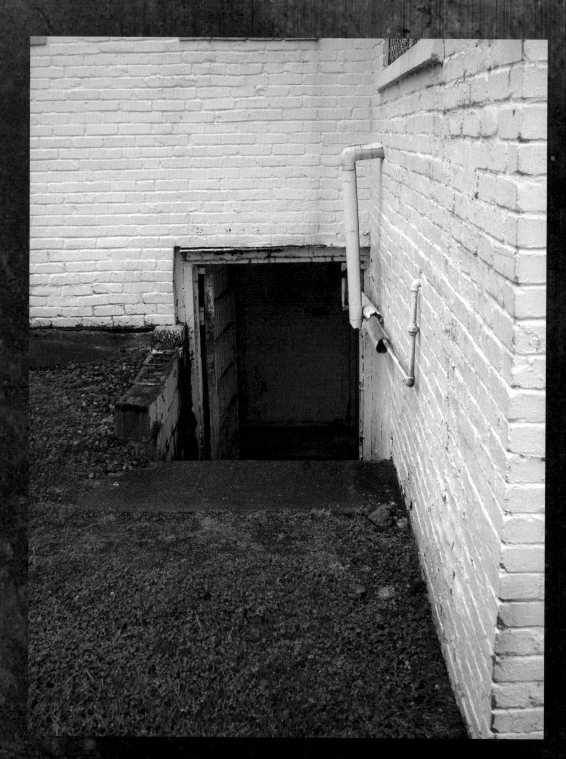

The entrance to the Sugar Shack. *Photo courtesy of the author.*

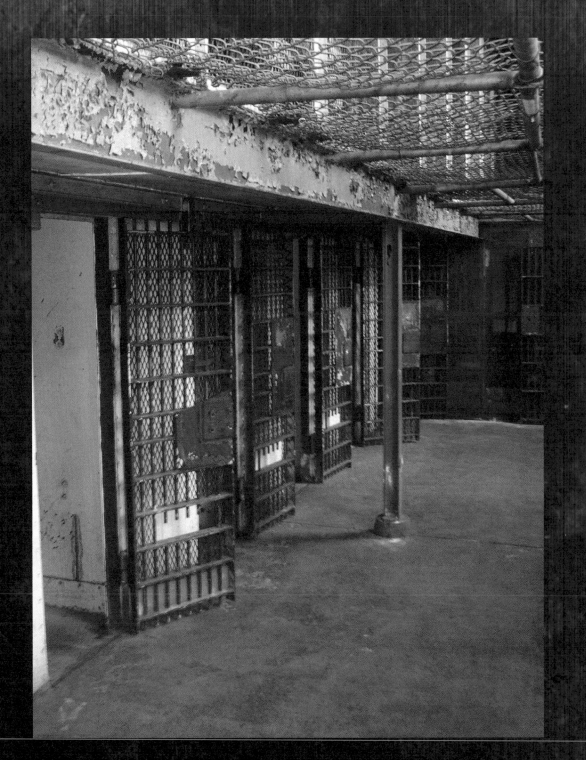

The maximum security cells in North Hall. "Red" Snyder spent twenty-two hours a day in the last cell on the left. Now, it is said he spends eternity there. *Photo courtesy of the author.*

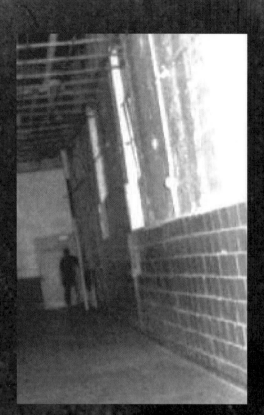

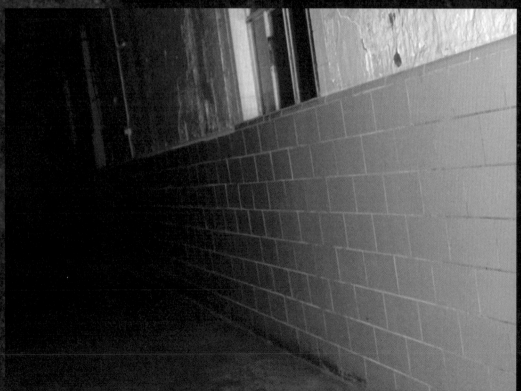

The North Hall, leading to the cafeteria door, where Polly Gear took the now-famous Shadow Man photograph. *Photo courtesy of Polly Gear.*

2.

WAVERLY HILLS SANATORIUM

Lousiville, Kentucky

1919-1982

"It is in moments of illness that we are compelled to recognize that we live not alone but chained to a creature of a different kingdom, whole worlds apart, who has no knowledge of us and by whom it is impossible to make ourselves understood: our body."

~Marcel Proust

Tuberculosis is a devastating disease. An airborne bacterial infection, it lodges itself deep inside the lungs, creating massive tumors that obstruct the airways and cause deep, choking fits of coughing, often resulting in blood-stained mucous clots. The pain is excruciating, the results devastating. If death does not take the TB patient, then the long-lasting damage it creates in its wake makes life miserable for those who survive it. This leads to the main difference between the hospital and the prison. In prison, convicts are punished and suffer involuntarily for their crimes, while those languishing in hospitals and asylums are there simply because they suffer and want to get well.

During the great tuberculosis epidemic of the '20s and '30s, treatment centers were few and far between. Hospitals filled up with TB patients quickly. In reaction, most every state began to cut funding to hospitals; they relocated those funds into the building of Tuberculosis clinics or hospitals, treatment centers that specialized specifically in the management of the tuberculosis bacteria. One of those hospitals was Waverly Hills Sanatorium.

The Sanatorium was built on the outskirts of Louisville, Kentucky, in 1911 by architects James J. Gaffney and Dennis X. Murphy. Serving the bulk of Jefferson County, the two-story building initially was built to accommodate only forty to fifty patients at a time. A year later, a second hospital for advanced cases was built, and still, in 1916, a children's wing was added, making the official hospital capacity at around 130 patients. Its architecture was revolutionary, constructed in a semi-circle so that the large open windows could catch as much fresh air and Vitamin rich sunlight for the ravaged health of the patients as possible.

Still, this was not enough. The onslaught of the so-called "White Plague" was ravaging the nation and plans were developed to construct a new building, one that stood five stories and would hold possibly up to 400 patients. Construction was complete in October of 1926. This is the structure that stands there today. It was a place of comfort for the many souls who dangled so helplessly near death. The Sanatorium had become their home, the other patients, their friends and neighbors. During its heyday, Waverly Hills meant hope and peace and comfort.

But no mistake was ever made when it was said that suffering abounded at Waverly Hills. During its run, estimates have ranged from 5,000 to 50,000 deaths attributed to tuberculosis. The end for these patients was hard and brutal, painful and shocking.

But as time went on, research revealed a powerful new antibiotic in the form of Streptomycin, and cases of tuberculosis lowered drastically, so drastically that a sanatorium the size of Waverly Hills was no longer cost effective enough to keep open. Patients were farmed out to the neighboring Hazelwood Sanatorium, and, by 1962, Waverly Hills had closed for good.

But its second incarnation, as Woodhaven Geriatrics Hospital, was far less comforting and genteel. Almost as soon as Waverly Hills reopened as Woodhaven Hospital, allegations of brutal abuse of the patients began to circulate. The elderly being housed there suffered severe bouts of neglect and physical and mental abuse, all at the hands of doctors, nurses, and orderlies. It closed in 1981 because of these allegations.

It stood empty and prone to vagrants and vandalism for years, the deed of ownership passing through many different hands. At one point, it was going to become a minimum security prison, and, later, an arts and worship center for the Christ The Redeemer Foundation. But these ideas fell through and Waverly Hills fell into disrepair.

Eventually, Waverly Hills was sold to Charlie and Tina Mattingly in 2001, and as late as 2008, there were plans to convert Waverly Hills into a four-star hotel. But the current owners have found much more success renting it out to paranormal investigators and conducting day and nighttime tours of Waverly Hills. They even host a haunted house attraction every Halloween with all proceeds going toward the property's restoration.

The Fourth Floor

Ask any paranormal investigator who has explored Waverly Hills which floor contains the most paranormal activity, and you will receive an almost unanimous answer. Investigators report more claims of footsteps, whispers, knockings and bangings, full-bodied apparitions, and clear-as-crystal EVPs on the fourth floor than on any other.

The fourth floor was used to house the sickest of the patients, with a majority of the more tedious and drastic surgeries being performed on that floor. In the midst of surgery, death can come quickly and leave the spirits anxious, confused, and unable to move on as they lament their former life.

To many, the air is heavier there, filled with a sadness, misery, and anguish that many find difficult to take. The sounds of the heavy doors slamming shut have been heard often, the sheer density of the doors assuring one that the wind—strong as it might be—could never slam the doors as violently as they had been slammed.

A story circulating through the Waverly Hills community is that of two young boys who broke into the abandoned hospital sometime in the 1990s, armed with spray paint and a hatchet, their intent being to vandalize the place beyond all recognition. They were discovered by security banging on the door that opens up onto the fourth floor. Their voices were loud and filled with terror as they begged the security guards for help. "The door's stuck! Get us out of here!" they'd screamed. But the security officers merely tugged the door open and the boys fell down the stairs onto the landing leading to the third floor. There were deep marks in the door from where one of the boys had used the hatchet to try and break the door down. Nothing worked. *Something* kept that door closed until the security guards opened it from the other side.

What had they seen? And more importantly, what was done to them to fill them with such terror and dread? Were the spirits of Waverly Hills tormenting the boys for vandalizing their home, for being inherently disrespectful? The boys refused to talk about it further, and one of them actually stepped up as a volunteer to help restore Waverly Hills in an effort to atone for his past misdeeds. But he still will not step foot inside the building.

Dark shapes dart through doorways, gliding through the hallways quickly, disappearing from one room and into another. Reactions from the spirits are mixed: some show interest in the living, while others ignore them completely and go about their business accordingly. This seemingly random series of encounters proves that what happens at Waverly Hills is the result of both Residual and Intelligent Hauntings. One thing that does appear certain is that there seems to be no ill will, hate, or animosity shown toward the living. Except perhaps from The Creeper...

Timmy and The Nurses of The Fifth Floor

The top floor of Waverly Hills has the distinction of having two reported suicides at Waverly Hills and, surprisingly, they were employees of the hospital. The first suicide supposedly occurred in 1928. According to most of the legends, the victim was a young nurse who had become pregnant without getting married. Devastated by the ostracism she was inevitably facing from her family and friends and growing increasingly despondent, the young nurse hung herself in room 502. This is one story.

Another story says that the young nurse had an affair with a doctor on staff at Waverly Hills and when she became pregnant, he performed a secret abortion on her. The nurse died on the operating table. Fearing that his reputation would suffer, he restaged her body in room 502, hanging her corpse from the ceiling. Supposedly, an aborted fetus was found floating in a deep cistern on the hospital grounds. Because the fifth floor was essentially a nurse and supply station at the time, it is possible that such things happened in relative privacy, especially during the nighttime hours.

The second incident happened in 1932 when a nurse allegedly threw herself from the rooftop patio and fell to her death. It is unclear why she chose to end her life, and the lack of any death records from the time seem to dispute whether the suicides happened at all.

However, whether these stories of nurse suicides are true or not, there is a presence in room 502. Apparitions seen there have been of a white draped figure, which could be the reason why so many people believe it is the spirit of a nurse or doctor. The dark silhouettes of men and women have been seen moving across the windows, blocking out the light from outside.

During Waverly Hills' time as a tuberculosis clinic, much of the fifth floor was open-aired, with serene patios and plenty of fresh air, as many patients flourished during sessions of "heliotherapy," therapy derived from the basking in sunlight. Direct sunlight was said to kill the tuberculosis bacteria, and the presence of Vitamin D can do further damage to the existing bacteria.

Because children benefited most from the effects of heliotherapy, playgrounds and open patios were installed on the roof so that the children could actually, and finally, enjoy themselves as they suffered their condition. It should come as no surprise, then, that the fifth floor roof contains the trapped souls of children who have passed on. Many visitors and employees of the estate report the eerie, distant echoes of nursery rhymes, and children playing have been heard often coming from these areas. These sounds could be signs of a Residual Haunting, yet, perhaps, they are signs of an intelligent one, as the spirits of the children return to the playgrounds they loved and continue to play on to this day.

One of those children seems to be the spirit of Timmy, who has been heard in various EVPs and continually participates in playtime with paranormal investigators who bring a rubber playground ball with them. The spirit of Timmy has been known to move the ball around in full view of investigators, though no real photographic proof of his apparition has ever been taken. But EVPs reveal the tiny laughter of a singular young boy, estimated in age perhaps of three or four years. Shadow figures supporting the playful specter back up the claims of Timmy, as pint-sized shades appear to investigators on occasion and try to lull them into a game of hide and seek.

Recently, Tina Mattingly, the owner of Waverly Hills, reopened a long sealed-off portion of Waverly Hills, the notorious Nurses' Wing. This Wing was dedicated to the Nurses who would contract tuberculosis during the course of their employ at Waverly Hills. It was a sad state to be in, but it was a selfless sacrifice these fine women made so that their patients could be well taken care of.

Dangerous structural damage prevented Tina from opening the wing up for tours, but as of October 2011, the damage has been repaired and the doors unsealed. Almost as soon as it was reopened, activity began. Intelligent responses in the form of loud knocks have answered "Yes" and "No" questions posed by investigators with ease.

It is also in the Nurses' Wing that a new specter has shown itself: "The Creeper."

Investigators will see what they believe to be a clump of shadows and think nothing of it...until the shadow stands up and reveals itself as a horrifying, humanoid black mass that escapes the curious by creeping up the walls and eventually disappearing into them. It moves quickly and casts a large pall over those fortunate enough to catch glimpses of it. The exact purpose of The Creeper's existence is unknown, as are its intentions. Further investigations, I am certain, will yield more evidence, more stories will arise, and The Creeper's legend will at some point flourish.

The Body Chute

The "Body Chute" is over 500 feet long, sloping down the base of a steep and treacherous hill and was used to bring supplies into the hospital. One side had steps for employees and delivery men to enter and exit the hospital without having to navigate the wooded and rough countryside. Mostly dark, save for a few skylights to provide a modicum of illumination and fresh air, it soon took on a different, more morose purpose.

At the peak of the tuberculosis epidemic, there could have been as many as fifty deaths per day at Waverly Hills. In an effort to keep the morale of the surviving patients up, doctors, nurses, and administrators transformed the tunnel into the Body Chute. Its purpose was singular and effective: provide a discrete pathway, away from patients eyes, for the exodus of all of the bodies leaving Waverly Hills. In its lifetime as the Body Chute, the tunnel saw the departure of thousands of bodies, and, according to numerous investigators and employees, still retains the massive amounts of negative energy expelled by the spirits.

This is one place in Waverly Hills that every paranormal investigator flocks to first. The experiences here are rather tame compared to the other parts of the building, but are unnerving all the same. Much of it can be attributed to the dense, thick atmosphere of claustrophobia. The walls seem to close in on you the further down the tunnel you go, and sometimes, the echo of footsteps behind you can add to the already overwhelming feelings of being watched in the darkness. Investigators have reported hearing whispers in the darkness and feeling the faint touch of ghostly fingers on their necks, hands, and faces as they struggle through the blackness.

The darkest entities swim in their sadness and search for peace in the last home they ever knew, surrounded by the last friends they ever loved. To many, Waverly Hills is a spirit-infested haunted place. But to the spirits themselves, it is their last and, for some, only home.

Psychic Impressions

Without a doubt, most every medium who has investigated Waverly Hills has encountered one singular spirit whose rage and anger tends to cast a pall over the former sanatorium and almost always pushes his way to the front of the line when the curious come to visit. In fact, it is his rage and anger that creates the darkness most people feel in Waverly Hills.

No one is sure what his name was, but back in the 1990s, a homeless man began to use the old Waverly Hills building as a shelter for himself and his beloved dog. He had been seen around the area a time or two with his white terrier, but few realized that he was squatting at the old hospital. Together, they would walk the seemingly endless halls until night fell and they huddled together for warmth in one of the interior rooms of the old clinic.

Just by sheer chance, a group of curious teenagers had wandered onto Waverly Hills and found the homeless man and his dog dead at the bottom of the elevator shaft. One might think that the man and his dog lost their way in the dark and simply fell down the shaft to their deaths. Not so, say the psychic mediums. All agree that they were thrown down the shaft, murdered in cold blood. The man was thrown in first, followed by the dog. News reports of the tragedy are scant, but police did eventually arrest a group of juveniles who confessed to the murder of the man and his dog. Because they were juveniles, their identities and the details of their exploits were kept from the media.

Now the homeless man stalks Waverly Hills, angry about being killed and enraged at those who trespass on the property he once considered his home.

Could this homeless man be the infamous Creeper spotted in the Nurse's Wing? Volunteers and tour guides at Waverly Hills told me personally that they have seen the ghost of the dog more often then that of the old man. The cute, white-haired dog will be seen curled up asleep on the floor. Then, as if roused from sleep, the dog will stand and walk away, vanishing into thin air. The dog has also been seen walking along the tree line behind the building, disappearing into the thick foliage.

Meditations on Waverly Hills brought me into contact with two people. The first was an old man clad in a hospital gown. He was gaunt, but not unhealthy. He stood by the Body Chute, looking about nervously. He called himself "Hardesty." Unlike many of the spirits at Waverly Hills, he did not die as a result of tuberculosis. Hardesty passed during Waverly Hills' time as a geriatric hospital. He did not speak a word to me, but made sure that I knew he was looking out for the shadow mass known as The Creeper. His fear frightened me.

Another soul I came into contact with was a nurse named Darla or Darlington, but I'm leaning toward Darla. She was on the fourth floor of the hospital waving to me. The words in my head came from her, most definitely: "We're waiting for you."

Meditation didn't come easy for me when I toured Waverly Hills in May 2012. In fact, it didn't come at all. Loud tour groups of forty made it difficult to connect with the spirits that I believe I had seen and come into contact with before. The spirits were there, but they were the tourists, not us. I could feel them watching us all as we made our way through the place, like some sort of demented zoo parade that we had stumbled into. Occasionally, I would see dark flashes from the corners of my eyes. I walked out of Waverly Hills without a single paranormal or spiritual connection. Hardesty and Darla were nowhere to be found, which bothered me because I truly wanted them to know I was there. Chances are, though, they already knew.

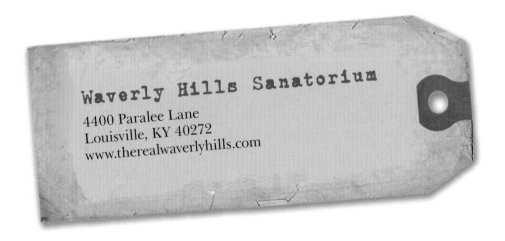

Waverly Hills Sanatorium

4400 Paralee Lane
Louisville, KY 40272
www.therealwaverlyhills.com

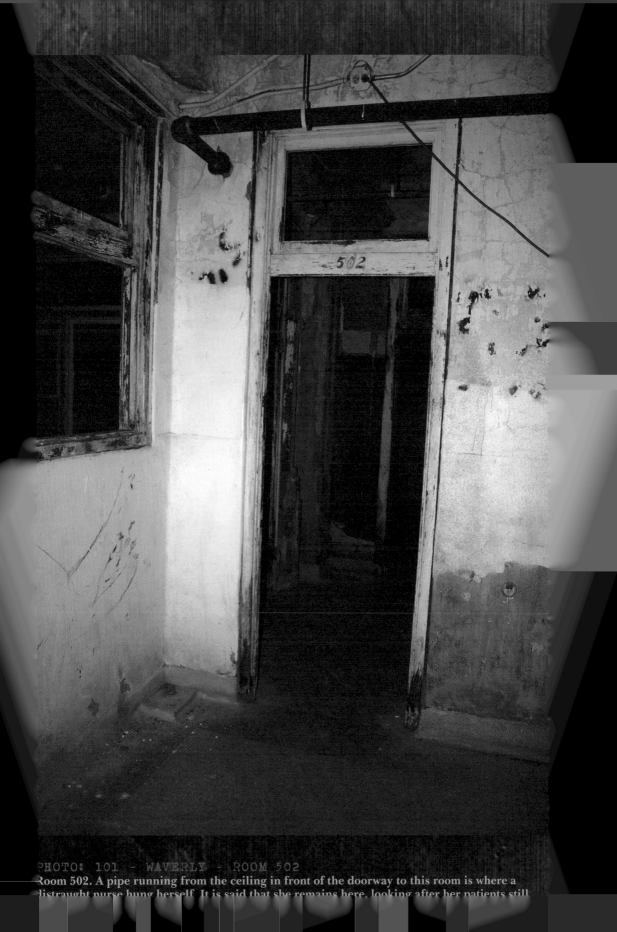

Room 502. A pipe running from the ceiling in front of the doorway to this room is where a distraught nurse hung herself. It is said that she remains here, looking after her patients still.

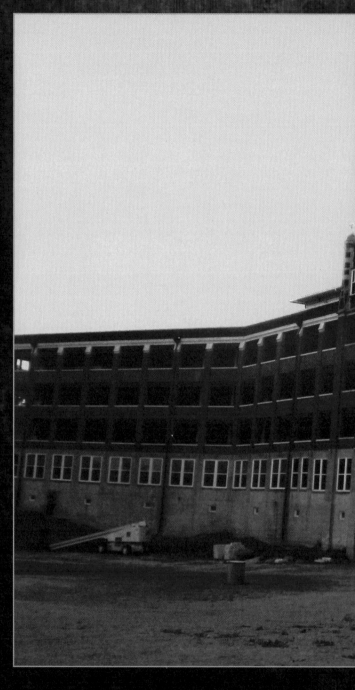

Waverly Hills Sanatorium. *Photo courtesy of the author.*

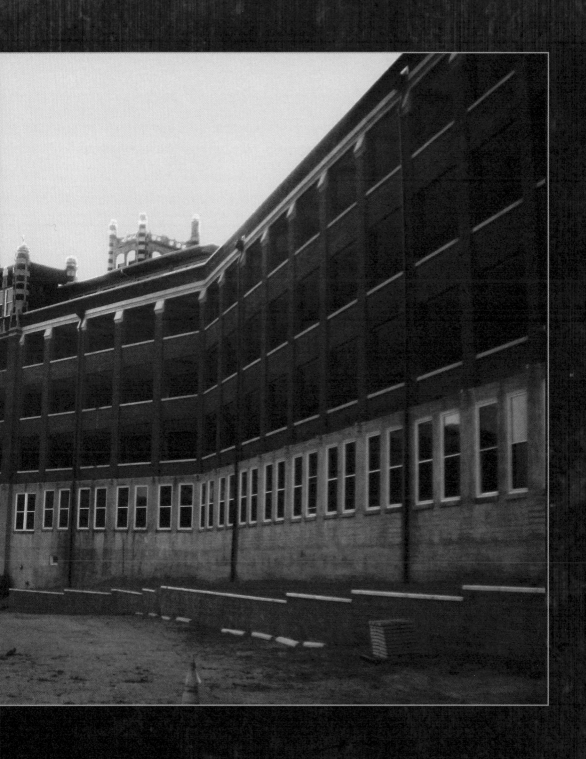

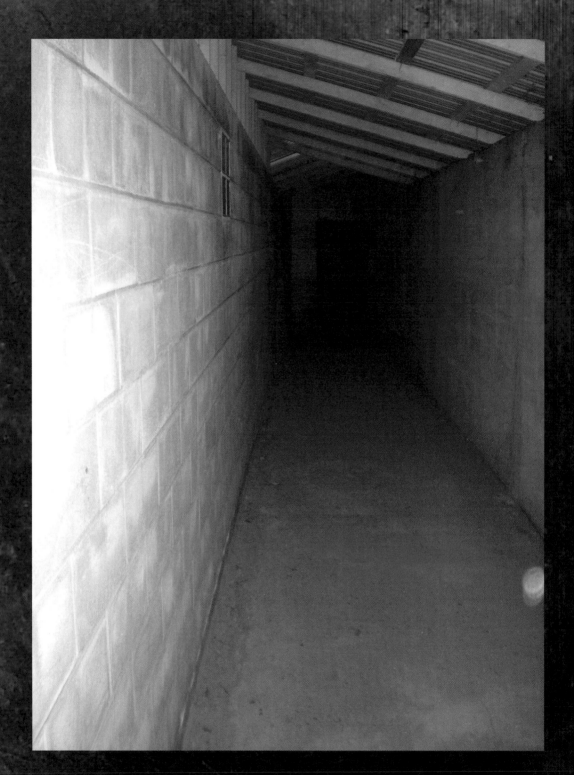

PHOTO 99 - WAVERLY - DEATH TUNNEL 2
The infamous Body Chute of Waverly Hills. *Photo courtesy of the author.*

3.

ANDERSONVILLE PRISON
Andersonville, Georgia

1864-1865

"Took a walk around camp. Deplorable sight. Some without clothing, some in last agonies
of death; others writhing under the pangs of disease or wounds; some as black as mulatttos
with smoke and dirt."

~Eugene Forbes
Sgt., Co. B, 4th New Jersey Infantry

It has been called America's Auschwitz, a death camp for Union prisoners
of war during the Civil War that began in 1861 and came to an end in 1865.
The treatment of the prisoners there rivaled anything that Adolph Hitler could
concoct in his quest to exterminate the Jews during World War II, and it is entirely
possible that Hitler used the example of Andersonville as a template for his
own cadre of concentration camps. Starvation, disease, epidemics of diarrhea,
murder, torture, and brutal and inhumane treatment were all ways in which the
Confederate army could exact their revenge against the Northern invaders. Even
though its capacity was estimated at just over 10,000 prisoners, it is believed that
over 45,000 prisoners were confined there during its run as the South's foremost
prison camp. Roughly 12,000 of those men perished because of the conditions.

Opened in February of 1864 as Camp Sumter, the prison lay in southwestern
Macon County, neighboring the east side of Andersonville, Georgia. Technically,
the prison lay in the small town of Americus, Georgia. It covered 16.5 acres and
a 15-foot-high stockade fence enclosed the entire camp. The prison camp was
overseen by Heinrich Hartmann Wirz, also known as Henry Wirz, a well-educated
Swiss immigrant with an established medical office in Louisiana when the Civil
War broke out. Entering the Confederate army as a private, he quickly rose to the
rank of Captain and assumed command of Camp Sumter in 1864.

Initially, there were plans to build wooden barracks, but Confederate officials
opted instead to leave the prison as an open-air stockade; it was, after all, only a
temporary prison for Union soldiers where they could be held in exchange for
Confederate prisoners captured by the North. The open-air conditions made it
necessary for the prisoners to build their own shelters, often using blankets and
sticks to create makeshift tents.

From the very beginning, food and medical rations were small, even
miniscule. Although a large amount of animosity between the North and South
could have been a deciding factor, it is decidedly more probable that the lack of
food and medical rations was due to the fact that the North had enacted a trade
blockade that left the Southern states unable to import or trade for their own
goods. These were situations that Captain Wirz could not control, but situations he

would be forced to atone for during his war crimes trial following the end of the Civil War.

In his own words, an anonymous Union soldier described his first impressions as he and his platoon of ninety soldiers were led into the prison for the first time:

> As we entered the place, a spectacle met our eyes that almost froze our blood with horror, and made our hearts fail within us. Before us were forms that had once been active and erect—stalwart men, now nothing but mere walking skeletons, covered with filth and vermin. Many of our men, in the heat and intensity of their feeling, exclaimed with earnestness. "Can this be hell?" "God protect us!" and all thought that He alone could bring them out alive from so terrible a place. In the center of the whole was a swamp, occupying about three or four acres of the narrowed limits, and a part of this marshy place had been used by the prisoners as a sink, and excrement covered the ground, the scent arising from which was suffocating. The ground allotted to our ninety was near the edge of this plague-spot, and how we were to live through the warm summer weather in the midst of such fearful surroundings, was more than we cared to think of just then.

Indeed, such a description only begins to describe the horrors inside Andersonville Prison, and prisoners would soon learn to fear not only their Confederate captors, but to fear rogue bands of Union soldiers out to make the best for themselves. One such group, calling themselves the Andersonville Raiders, regularly terrorized their fellow soldiers, robbing their shoes, jewelry, and clothes, even murdering them in order to get their hands on their meager, yet valuable, food rations.

Another rogue group arose to combat the Raiders, calling themselves The Regulators. They were able to subdue nearly all of the Raiders and brought them before Confederate judge Pete McCollough. They were all found guilty. Six of the Raiders were hanged, while the rest were made to suffer various forms of humiliating torture, such as being put into the Stocks and being forced to wear a ball and chain.

Finally, with the deaths of almost 13,000 prisoners under their belts, Camp Sumter was shut down at the end of the Civil War in 1865. Henry Wirz was taken into custody and court-martialed on charges of conspiracy and murder. He was the only Confederate to be brought up on charges of war crimes, only because he refused to implicate Confederate President Jefferson Davis, or any other of his superior officers.

Perhaps the most damning pieces of evidence at Wirz's trial was the detailed records by which the Confederacy tallied the enemy dead. At Andersonville, that duty was left to a Union prisoner named Dorence Atwater, who made a copy of the death records and had it published in the newspapers following the war. Of the 12,913 deaths at Andersonville, only 460 of them were listed in the logs as "unknown." To the War Crimes Tribunal, every murder that Wirz was accused of now had a name and a body to go with it. In the aftermath of such a bloody and vehement war, Wirz never stood a chance in the arena of Northern public opinion.

Wirz assumed all responsibility for Andersonville Prison and was found guilty. Sentenced to hang, his execution took place in Washington, D.C. on land that would soon become home to the Supreme Court of the United States.

The scars of Andersonville still pulsate to this day and the mere mention of it brings to mind the horrors of the worse behavior possible by mankind at his worst. It is this raw, negative energy that feeds the ghosts of Andersonville and keeps alive the memory that these restless spirits need to keep alive, for even they realize that if you do not remember the past, you are condemned to repeat it.

The Sounds and Smells of Death

The most reported, and most overwhelming, phenomena surrounding Andersonville Prison is the rising of an incredibly acrid smell that reminded one Vietnam veteran of a military field hospital. The smell of rotting corpses, bacterial infections, feces and urine, and of stagnant water oftentimes fill the grounds of the former prison turned National Monument.

Indeed, the smell of death was incredibly overpowering during the operation of the prison, even becoming a defining characteristic. It has been said that this smell was often accompanied by an unearthly fog that hid the silent specters of men in and out of uniform, moving in and out of the fog banks, disappearing at random. The appearance of the fog and the smells of the prison often correlate to certain anniversaries of note, such as the day Wirz was hanged and the day Andersonville was liberated. It has also been reported that sometimes, in the dead of night, Confederate soldiers can be seen walking the roads toward the prison, though stories of full-bodied apparitions of Confederates need to be taken with a grain of salt; Civil War re-enactors are famous for camping in the surrounding areas and going on "patrols" as part of their duty as said re-enactors.

Even more strange are the reports of sounds, such as the haunting sounds of gunfire, the heartbreaking screams of the dying, and the moans of agony. These sounds swirl about the place, radiating all over, so that one cannot pinpoint with any degree of accuracy where they are originating from. But in the night, does it really matter where the screams originate? The fact that you hear them at all is enough to make your blood curdle.

Many of these re-enactors, especially the ones who don garb as Confederates, are targeted specifically by the ghosts of Andersonville. They are the first to smell the stench of death and filth. They will be the first to hear the screams of dying men, and see the specters of dead men in their ghostly fog. Perhaps it is their way of showing their Confederate captors how much they suffer still.

Father Whelan

During the year it was open for business as a prison, an Irish Catholic cleric named Father Peter Whelan ministered faithfully to the captives of Andersonville, earning the nickname "The Angel of Andersonville" from the prisoners who loved him. He had even brought clothing, food, and money from nearby Savannah, prompting one Union soldier to declare that, "without a doubt, he was the means of saving hundreds of lives."

And he appears to still be ministering to the restless dead of Andersonville, for the spirit of a priest, garbed in his Catholic robes, has been seen on the prison grounds, as well. There were two priests assigned to Andersonville, Father Whelan and Reverend William Hamilton. While Hamilton was repelled by the sight of the Union prisoners covered in lice and dying from dysentery and starvation, and never commingled with the prisoners, Whelan saw thousands of souls in need of faith and hope. His kind nature and gentle demeanor earned him much respect and love from the doomed prisoners. When the Civil War came to a close in 1865, Father Whelan appeared and gave favorable testimony to prosecutors on behalf of Captain Wirz. Eventually, Whelan returned to Savannah, and headed up St. Patrick's Church until his death from tuberculosis in 1868.

Although his tenure was limited to only four months, eyewitnesses claim that the specter of the priest most resembles Father Whelan, who makes his rounds amongst the devoted who count on his aid and faith to get them through their own personal Hells.

Some investigators have not only seen Father Whelan, but have heard his voice as well, such as the story of historian Robert Berry, a writer who used the topic of Andersonville as his master's thesis. Berry was walking the grounds during the waning hours of the afternoon just as it was about to give way to night. He began to smell the familiar stench of death and saw a strange figure walking ahead of him, a figure who seemingly vanished into the night air. Berry then heard the voice of a man coming from behind him, saying, "I'm going to give him the last rites." When Berry turned, he found himself staring into the face of a Catholic priest he claims was Father Whelan. Upon uttering those chilling words, the visage of Whelan faded from view and disappeared.

Since its closure in 1865, Andersonville Prison has become a National Historic Place, recognized as such in 1970. Today, it encompasses a cemetery for the dead and a prisoner of war museum, as well as a finely preserved representation of the prison stockade itself. To gaze upon it, you can't help but feel the misery of the past seep into the present, burrowing into your soul, just as the restless phantoms of Andersonville would like.

Andersonville National Historic Site

496 Cemetery Road
Andersonville, GA 31711

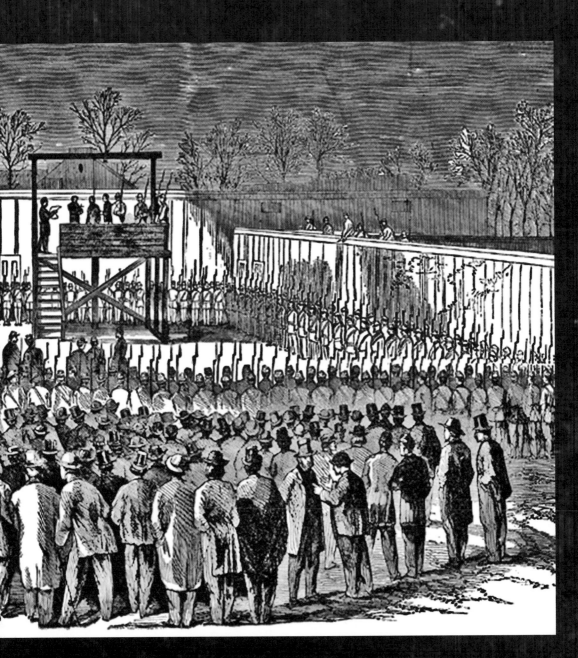

PHOTO 58-WIRZ EXECUTION ILLUSTRATION
An 1865 illustration detailing the public execution of Captain Henry Wirz.

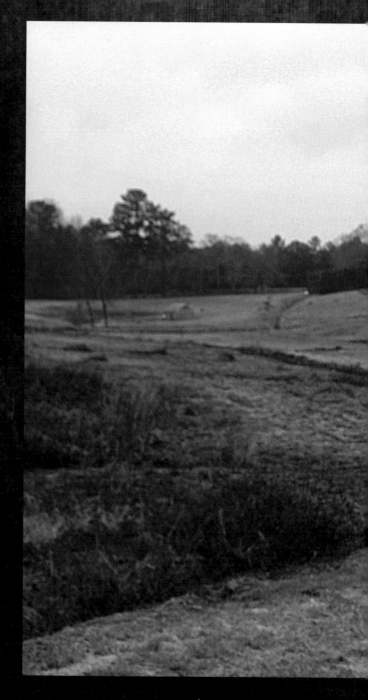

PHOTO 33: ANDERSONVILLE SINKS

This stream in the Andersonville prison camp was the Union Prisoner of War's only source of fresh water. It was also used as a sink and toilet. *Photo courtesy of Robert Schoenman.*

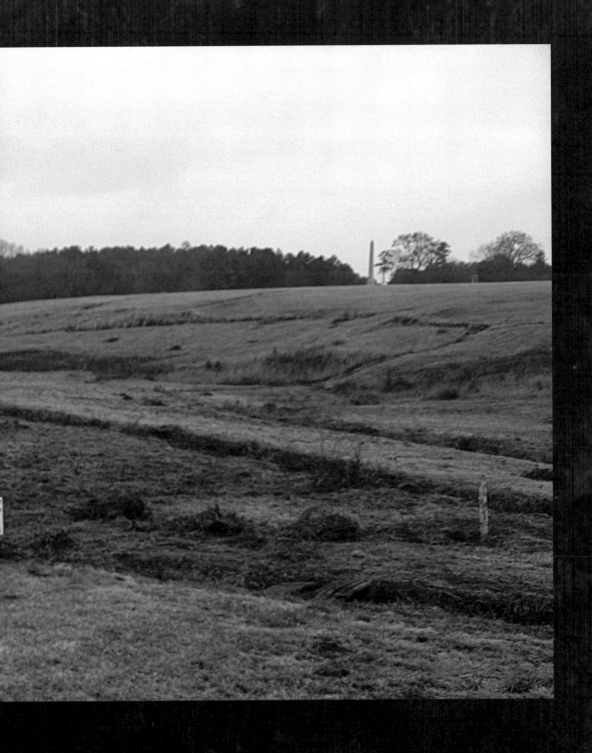

43

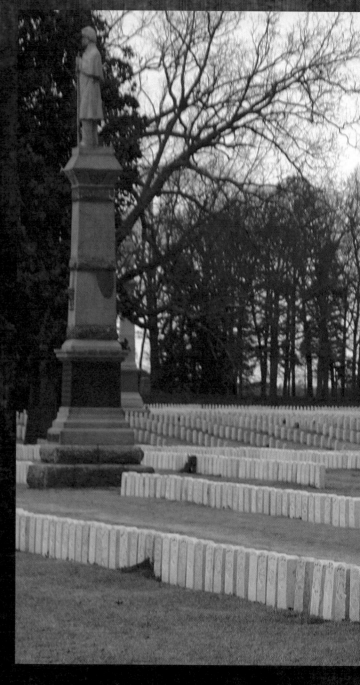

PHOTO 32-ANDERSONVILLE CEMETERY
The cemetery of Andersonville today. *Photo courtesy of Robert Schoenman.*

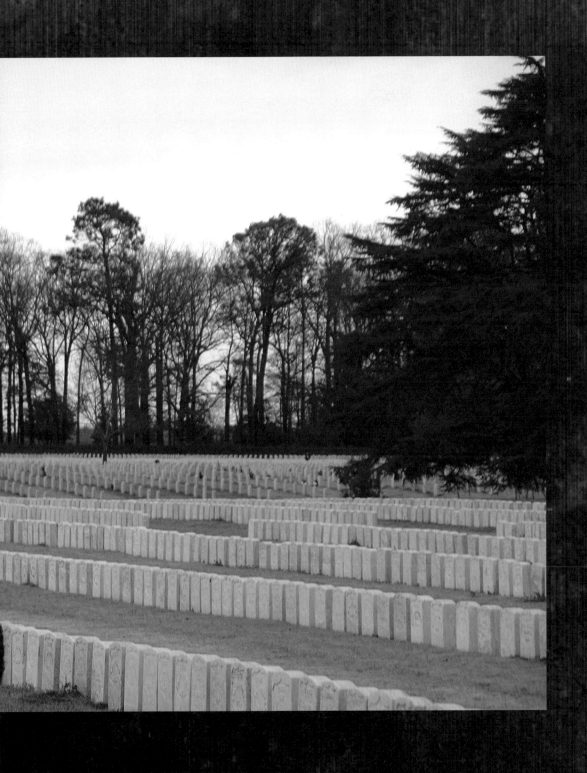

4.

THE ASYLUMS OF NEW JERSEY

"We do not have to visit a madhouse to find disordered minds; our planet is the mental institution of the universe."

~Goethe

The Abandoned Village of Ancora Psychiatric Hospital
Verona, New Jersey

Driving south on Route 30, you'll see the signs for it. Most pass by, but for those with time on their hands and a curious nature, it is an invitation. In this spot in Verona, New Jersey, sat a hundred homes that have now been demolished and carted away. Save for a few buildings used as storage and the eerie line of working streetlights, no one would guess that there once stood a thriving tract of subdivision homes. The roads, once paved and deeply black, have been stripped away, replaced by mud and decades-old tire ruts that cut through the underbrush like a frontier trail. This village, used as lodging for the hospital employees, has become an urban ghost town that swells with the past lives of tortured souls and the broken dreams they clung tightly to in the night. It is an eerie mirror to the souls lost in the psychiatric hospital directly across the street.

Built in 1955, this abandoned village was constructed by the state and run by the Ancora Psychiatric Hospital as a town for their employees where community banquets, flea markets, sporting events, swimming pools, and tiny shops were highlights of a golden age. Located across from the Ancora Psychiatric Hospital, it provided a perfect location at bare-bones pricing for the employees of Ancora and their families.

However, a budget crisis cut funding to the hospital and rent amongst the employees rose dramatically, leading to a mass exodus of tenants from the homes. The state attempted to compensate their losses by lending them out to various state agencies as low income or transitional housing. By the time 1988 rolled around, drug dealers and murderers roamed the neighborhood. This was the new age of crack, that devastating cocaine-based drug that took the world by the throat throughout the '80s and '90s. Gang wars, drug wars, burglaries, muggings, murders, suicides, and prostitution would have run rampant in this subdivision as the drug dealers staked their claims, made their money, destroyed their competitors, and enslaved hundreds of addicts. Hospital security, still in charge of policing the area, found themselves patrolling a war zone. Finally, as violence rose and blood was spilled, the state stepped in, bulldozing the homes and closing the village for good. Now, with the exception of only a few shack-like homes, there is no evidence that the once-beloved suburb of Ancora Psychiatric Hospital was even there at all.

Still, there is life thriving in the woods once home to over 100 manufactured homes. Shadowy figures have been spotted moving amongst the trees late at night, and loud whispers have been heard in some of the few buildings that actually remain.

One story tells of a woman being chased by a black shadow figure as she fled one of the remaining buildings. She responded to a message on my Wyandotte Paranormal Society Facebook page when I asked if anyone had tales to tell of haunted prisons or asylums. Because the art of urban exploration is frowned upon by law enforcement, she asked to remain anonymous, but shared her tale nonetheless.

Her boyfriend was a self-described "urban explorer," an adventurer type who typically sneaked into abandoned buildings in order to explore them. She tagged along with him when he had decided to explore what remained of the abandoned village at Ancora. Once inside one of the few remaining buildings, the couple was startled by incoherent whispers coming from another room. As the whispers grew louder, the woman realized that some of the darkness in the house was actually moving. Genuinely frightened, the woman fled when the shadow figure suddenly darted toward her.

There is no real way to validate the woman's statement. Most all of the buildings, sidewalks, and paved roads were destroyed, the debris trucked away as the woods began to reclaim the former property. But some shack-like homes and barns still remain, used for storage for the hospital across the street, and it is possible that it was one of these buildings our storyteller and her boyfriend happened upon. In any case, because it is owned by the state and requires permission, very little legal evidence of paranormal activity exists. But word of mouth amongst employees and those brave enough to risk arrest by trespassing return to the real world with tales of a spooky, supremely creepy ghost town.

Across the street from the abandoned village of Ancora is the main psychiatric hospital, Ancora Psychiatric Hospital. The most notorious branch of this hospital is the one reserved for those who have been deemed "criminally insane," mentally unbalanced murderers, rapists, child molesters, and deranged schizophrenics who have been found not guilty because of their obvious insanity. Two sets of fences and a massive army of armed guards keep escape attempts to a minimum.

But in 2007, William Enman, a paranoid schizophrenic with a history of brutal violence against adults and children alike, escaped from one of the buildings at Ancora that was surrounded by a fence only eight feet high. Authorities searched as far as Canada before Enman was found still on hospital grounds. Another escapee named Dewitt Crandall, Jr., who had killed his mother and father with a hunting knife in 1996, simply walked off the grounds. He was found one town over near the railroad tracks, stark naked, and returned to Ancora Psychiatric. Admitted to the infirmary for observation, Crandall, Jr. eventually hanged himself with a bed sheet in one of the hospital restrooms.

Because this facility is still in operation and the security surrounding it is super tight, not too many stories have surfaced about whether or not there are any hauntings onsite. But a few rumors have managed to creep out from the mouths of former employees who report strange whispers in the shower rooms, as well as faint shadows coursing through the hallways. Whether you choose to believe in the supposed hauntings at Ancora Psychiatric Hospital or not, it cannot be denied that it is an amazing location with an incredible history that lends itself quite well to urban legend and tales of the fantastic.

Greystone Park
Psychiatric Hospital
Morris Plains, New Jersey

Greystone Psychiatric Hospital, formerly known by the warmer and fuzzier name as the New Jersey State Lunatic Asylum, opened its doors on August 17, 1876. Its 30 buildings sat on over 700 acres, and when it opened, it was estimated that only about 600 patients could be housed comfortably. Exercise rooms, attic space, and lounge areas were converted into dormitories capable of housing the massive influx of patients seen from the late 1880s to the 1960s. Even folk singer Woody Guthrie "enjoyed" a stay at Greystone from 1956 to 1961, visited at one time by his number one fan, a man named Robert Zimmerman, who would later become very well known as Bob Dylan. It was Guthrie who nicknamed Greystone "Gravestone."

By that time, the population of the asylum had reached its peak with over 6,000 patients. But years of overcrowding, under funding, and negligence by maintenance staff made the governor of New Jersey declare Greystone to be irreparable and ordered it closed in 2003.

Reports of ghostly happenings in Greystone are rare, but an occasional eerie tale has risen from the decrepit hallways of the once imposing Kirkbride building. Like many of its Kirkbride counterparts, Greystone sports a series of tunnels running underneath the hospital connecting the various buildings and wings in a way that made transporting patients discreet and swift. Loud knocks and bangs have been heard in these tunnels, as have the sounds of hospital gurneys and far-off, disembodied moans.

Perhaps the most famous tale deals with a patient who tried to escape using the tunnels and was subsequently shot to death by guards in those very tunnels. His ghost is said to walk there still, wandering around the darkness. In other parts of the building, it was eerie, but not rare, to see unexplained light anomalies, full-bodied apparitions of patients and nurses, doors and windows opening on their own, and, perhaps most haunting of all, see the ghosts of former patients at the windows, still looking out, still seeing beyond the fences, still trying to see their freedom.

Essex County Hospital
Cedar Grove, New Jersey

Of all of New Jersey's haunted and abandoned asylums, it is the Essex County Hospital that has retained the title of most haunted and most famous. Also known as the Overbrook Asylum for the Insane and erected in 1872, Essex County Hospital was built specifically to house both hardcore criminals and moderately disturbed individuals. All who passed through the doors of Essex County Hospital suffered a mental distress that was etched into their faces until the day they died in their cells. It has been estimated that over 10,000 patients saw the end of their lives here and for some, their lives still go on, still full of sadness, still full of anger, still full of confusion.

Essex County Hospital saw its greatest tragedy in the winter of 1917 when the boilers failed and shut down, plunging the hospital into a maelstrom of freezing cold. Before help could arrive to repair the boilers, twenty people had frozen to death and thirty others suffered serious cases of frostbite.

Several different buildings make up the campus of Essex County Hospital and paranormal activity has been reported in each and every one of them. According to various paranormal groups that have investigated at the hospital, all report several instances of random cold spots and disturbing shadow figures in the labyrinthine underground tunnels. The sudden appearance of irregular, mist-like orbs have shown up in photographs taken inside, and the specter of a nurse has been spotted walking the hallways, still checking on her patients more than a century after her death.

But it is the dramatic, yet mundane, voices that echo throughout the hospital. Anything from intelligent responses to questions asked during investigations, to somewhat boring conversations between two or three different spirits, all heard with the naked ear and not as an EVP.

Sadly, Essex County Hospital is no more. The buildings were demolished by the State of New Jersey and re-dedicated as a wildlife reservation full of hiking trails and protected wildlife.

What was most apparent about the hospital was the incredible wave of sadness and sorrow that washed over you as you stepped inside. People who walked in made of brick walked out as a pile of jelly, with overwhelming feelings of melancholy still tugging at their souls to this day.

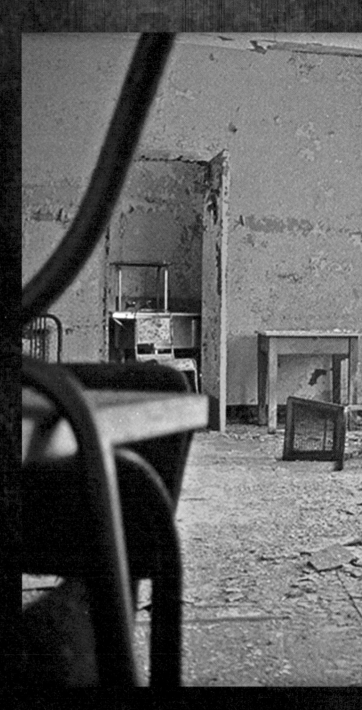

Photo courtesy of Kevin Husta, Owl's Flight Photography.

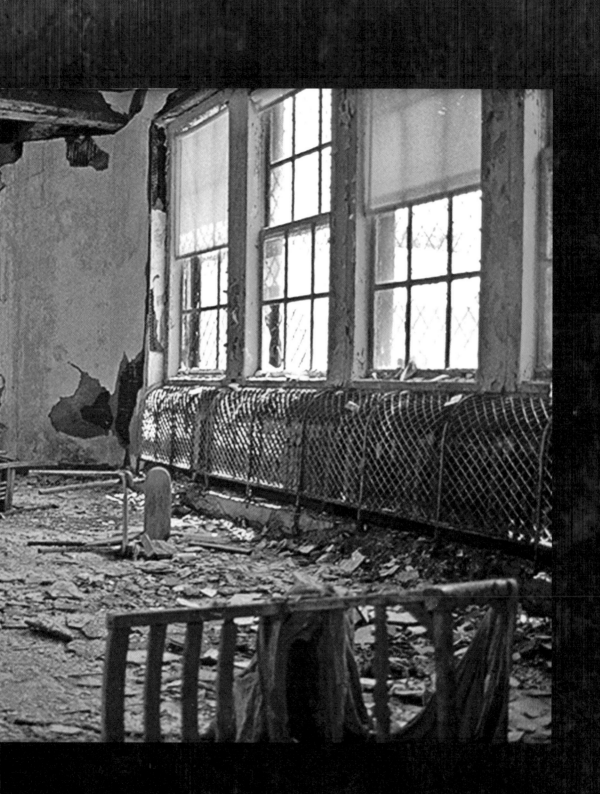

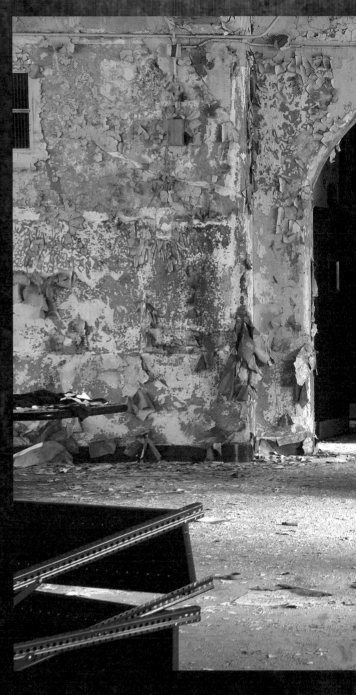

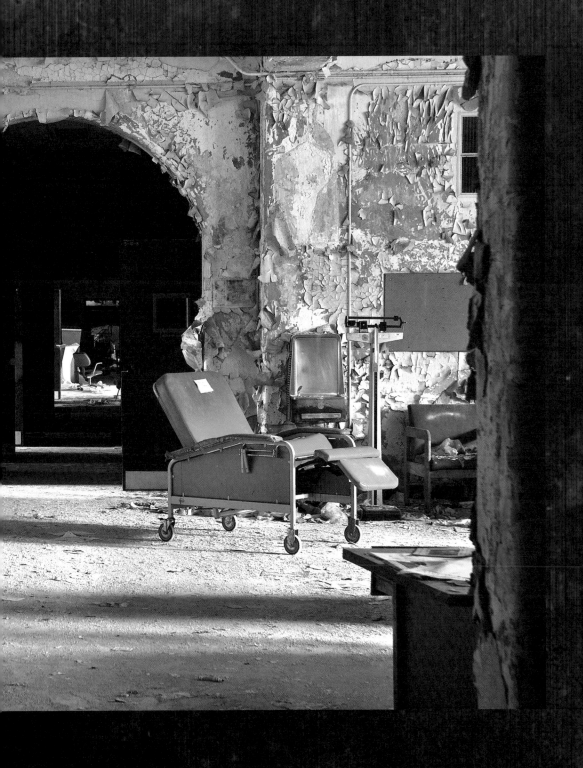

5.

ROLLING HILLS ASYLUM

Genesee County, New York

1827-1974

"Habitual drunkards, lunatics (one who by disease, grief, or accident lost the use of reason or from old age, sickness or weakness was so weak [sic] of mind as to be incapable of governing or managing their affairs), paupers (a person with no means of income), state paupers (one who is blind, lame, old, or disabled with no income source) or a vagrant."
~Directive by New York State government regarding the Genesee County Poorhouse, 1824

The above directive was drafted by New York State legislators in 1824, and charged that all counties within the state were to care for their poor, including finding property in which to house them. The properties had to have acreage for farming and be self sufficient. In 1826, Genesee County purchased 200 acres between Rochester and Buffalo, and got to work.

When the Genesee County Poorhouse was opened for business in January of 1827, the above list was printed in the Batavia newspapers, proclaiming who was eligible for service at the brand new facility. But over time, the list would change to include everyone from alcoholics to homosexuals to the mentally retarded. Eventually, anyone who was considered a burden would become eligible for the Poorhouse. Even a Farmer's widow would be placed here because women were never allowed to own property. "If you were a mother with children, you would be put on the same floor as drunkards and pedophiles," says paranormal investigator Stacey Jones. "This was considered the worst in the state as far as treatment to their residents."

Built in 1826, the 53,000 square-foot building sat upon over 200 acres and was a virtually self-sufficient, working farm. As time went on, and as needs grew, more buildings were built and incorporated onto the original structures. Residents would work the farm, raising cattle, swine, horses, and chickens. There was a carpentry shop and bakery, allowing residents to build and bake goods to sell in town. It was, for all intent and purposes, a small, very fertile town inside of another small town. Only *this* town was populated with the dregs of society, those nobody wanted. Those people others wanted to forget. Over the course of sixty years, the population became more dangerous as murderers and criminals were moved into the rank and file of the general population. Children of all ages, races, and sexes would be sold to farmers, salesmen, and others for cheap slave labor. Because of this, the State built new cells in the existing building, maximum security cells that would house these dangerous criminals. The Genesee County Poorhouse was now an asylum and prison.

In 1887, the state agreed to move all those suffering from "acute insanity" to other institutions, returning the Genesee County Poorhouse to its more focused beginnings as a workhouse for the county. This continued on unabated until the 1950s when the Poorhouse became a home for the elderly almost exclusively. By then, all of the former residents had been moved out of the Poorhouse and into a more suitable institution. In 1974, the facility was shut down and all of the residents relocated.

Twenty years passed and the Poorhouse stood empty. The cemetery beyond the gates was reclaimed by the forest, its headstones disappearing into the dark soil and tall grass. The building began to fall into disrepair.

Then, in 1992, the building reopened as Carriage House, housing several different boutique shops. It was then that the odd goings on were finally noticed. Patrons at the shops reported their clothing being tugged, hearing disembodied voices and screams, and intense feelings of being watched.

In 2002, the property was bought by Jeff and Lori Carlson, who renamed it Rolling Hills Country Mall. Although the mall is closed now, the Carlsons continued to live on the property in one of the outbuildings they had converted into a four bedroom home. In 2004, they began conducting ghost tours.

The legend of Rolling Hills, the haunted asylum, had begun. As interest in the old Poorhouse grew, thanks to word of mouth between paranormal groups, the old history and stories of its residents began to filter back into the present day, lost no longer. Now, the haunting had a purpose, the spirits had a name, and dark tales of patient and inmate abuse were about to become part of Bethany, New York's folklore.

Roy Crouse

Rolling Hills' most famous resident is said to be the spirit of Roy, a gentle man who they say suffered from gigantism, a condition in which the head, arms, legs, and fingers all grow at exponential rates. Born March 4, 1890, Roy Crouse was the son of a fairly prominent banker in Syracuse, about 115 miles east of the Poorhouse. Already fairly tall for his age, Roy's father dumped him at the Genesee County Poorhouse in 1902 when he was 12 years old; it is theorized that, as Roy Crouse entered puberty, his gigantism began to take off dramatically, so dramatically, in fact, that Roy's freakish height, distended arms and fingers, and enlarged head made it difficult for his family and neighbors to accept him.

Tragic as it may sound, this practice of abandoning your handicapped, retarded, or deformed children to the poorhouses and asylums of the world was an accepted facet in nearly every class of American society.

At the peak of his height, Roy Crouse stood well over seven feet tall, a hulking giant of a man whose arms and fingers hung low, perhaps almost to his knee caps. Roy was a favorite patient at the Poorhouse, truly living up to the term of "gentle giant." He was a self-educated man who spent his time alone in the library, pouring over books and filling his brain with the works of famous composers of the classical genre. Because of his incredible size, Roy was most likely left alone by the more bullying-type of orderly and nurse, but his reputation was one of soft-spoken gentleness. The Poorhouse was his home, a place where he was accepted and treated exceptionally well from the time he stepped foot inside.

Roy stayed at the home for fifty years, passing away at the age of 62, a relatively old age for someone enduring the effects of gigantism. A benign soul, Roy is said to walk the halls of Rolling Hills and has been photographed several times as a tall shadow figure. His deep voice has been captured numerous times, answering questions intelligently and thoughtfully. Roy tends to look after the asylum by showing an active interest in who is wandering about his home and he speaks easily to those he likes and trusts. Try using opera music as a trigger object; it was Roy's favorite kind of music.

Nurse Emmie and Raymond

If Roy was the gentlest soul at Rolling Hills, then Nurse Emmie Altworth would commonly be known as the nastiest. Notorious in her position as a caregiver for being violent, abusive, and negligent, Nurse Emmie had little patience for her wards and succeeded only in terrorizing them with her physical and verbal assaults.

She was the head nurse of the Poorhouse, doling out punishments not only to the inmates and patients, but also to other staff members lower on the seniority totem pole. It has been said that the rotation of nurses working under Emmie Altworth was constantly in flux and change. Not many could stomach working under her for long.

It has been speculated that Emmie was a more than proficient witch, a member of a coven that practiced black magic as opposed to the more benevolent Wicca (or White) magic. It is said that when she brought the coven into Rolling Hills and began performing rituals there, that the darkness already surrounding the asylum grew heavier and more impenetrable. If rituals were performed, a doorway would have been opened and spirits of all natures and personalities would have come through in droves, spirits from all corners of the earth, not just former residents of Rolling Hills.

When Nurse Emmie died, sightings of her ghost were immediate, especially around the third floor of the West Wing and the café area, where people would catch sight of an older woman walking the hallway toward the restrooms. Her presence, negative energy and all, has been felt in the infirmary wing, as well as in her apartment near the fourth floor. Massive blasts of icy air, accompanied by scratches, punches, and pushes are all considered her calling cards. Men, in particular, are favorite victims of hers, suffering the most abuse at her spectral hands, especially when provoked.

Raymond, meanwhile, seems to be Emmie Altworth's male counterpart. The nasty spirit of a former patient, Raymond was known to be a handful while he was alive. He was belligerent to the staff, abusive to his fellow patients, and was even thought to have sexually assaulted some of the female patients at Rolling Hills and molested some of the children.

His spirit, they say, is just as nasty.

Male investigators have been pushed and punched, while female investigators have actually been groped and gotten the feeling that a strong male presence was straight up in their faces. He stalks the basement and furnace rooms, much like he did in life, still waiting for someone to make a wrong turn and fall into his web. He rarely backs down from a challenge, and will do whatever is necessary to get what he wants.

The Screaming Woman

Her voice echoes throughout the Poorhouse, cutting through the light and the dark like a bullet, chilling your blood and stiffening your spine. It comes from out of nowhere, reaching into your soul and paralyzing it with horror. Of all of the phenomena at Rolling Hills, the most chilling and terrifying seems to be that of "The Screaming Woman."

Her name eludes us, but she has the scream of an old woman, shrill, raspy, and bloodcurdling, sounding as real and as clear as a human voice. Many people have reported hearing these screams, including Stacey Jones. "We were here not even five minutes and we heard it," she says. "It sounded like a blood curdling scream. I took off running because I was convinced somebody was here. It was that loud."

Indeed, in a place that housed people from the destitute to the thoroughly deranged, it would seem that screaming was one of the only ways they were able to communicate with their nurses, doctors, and fellow patients. Whether it be night or day, summer or winter, investigators, visitors, and volunteers alike all profess to hearing The Screaming Woman from time to time, and it always sends shivers racing down their backs, no matter how often her voice is heard screaming for help.

The Christmas Room

The forgotten patients of Rolling Hills were the vast numbers of children left there by their parents because they could either no longer afford to care for them, or they had been orphaned because of disease or some other kind of tragedy. A tragic situation, to be sure, but one that the people of Rolling Hills tried to make better by creating "The Christmas Room." Filled with artifacts, novelties, and decorations, The Christmas Room was a comforting place where the children could go, a place where it was always Christmas.

Chilling now and very creepy, the souls of those children return to The Christmas Room regularly, enjoying the toys they played with in life. Whether it be the invisible hands making the rocking horse move, or the colorful play balls and Matchbox cars being rolled across the floors, The Christmas Room is rife with paranormal activity. The voices of children, footsteps, and distant laughter have been heard, not only as EVPs, but with investigators' own ears.

But could the sound of children be a lure for human souls from something far removed from the soul of a child? That idea has been spoken aloud more than once by more than a few very reputable investigators, that the demonic force that seems to loom large over Rolling Hills is masquerading as a troop of ghost children in an attempt to entice naïve souls under its leathery wings. One may not open themselves up to a demon, but they will to a tragic ghost child searching for its mommy. Whether this is true or not is pure speculation and one that cannot be proven easily. But what can be said is that ghost children are not prone to emitting such feelings of dread, horror, and actual physical attacks such as punching and scratching. All of these traits are demonic in nature and not in the character of the spirits of children.

For now, Rolling Hills Asylum seems to be comfortable with what it is, as are its residents, who wander the halls still and share their home with a darkness they cannot escape, even in death.

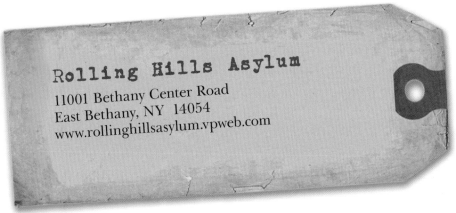

Rolling Hills Asylum
11001 Bethany Center Road
East Bethany, NY 14054
www.rollinghillsasylum.vpweb.com

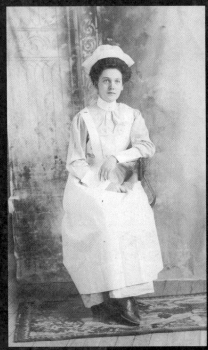

PHOTO: 69 - NURSE PORTRAIT
This is what the infamous Nurse
Emmie Altworth would have worn as
she tended to her patients.

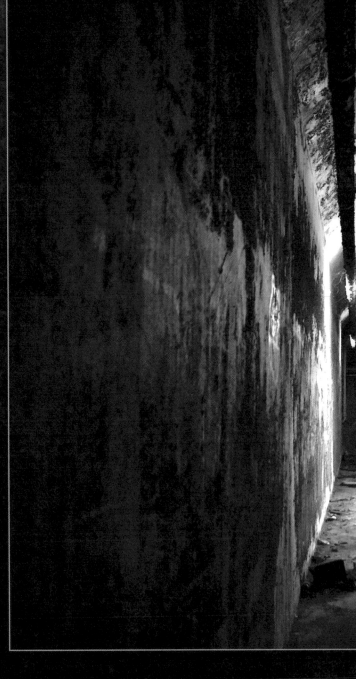

PHOTO: 107
Photo courtesy of Kevin H., Owl's Flight Photography.

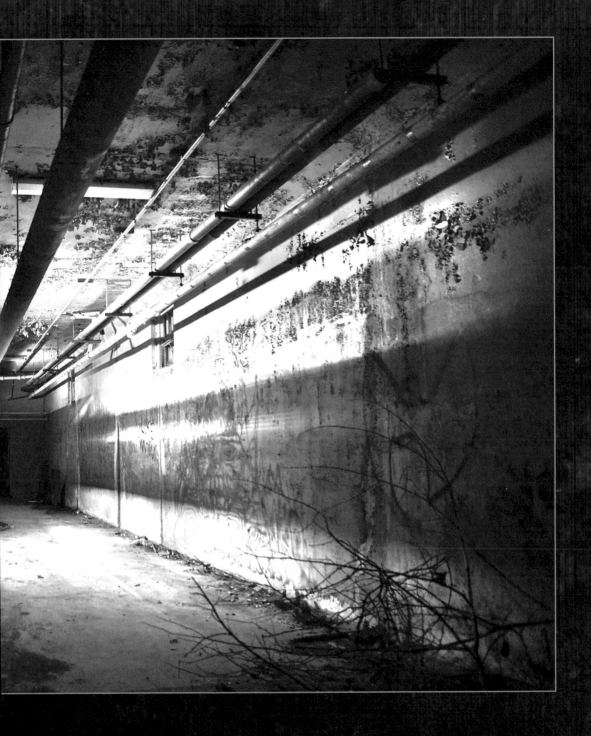

6.

DANVERS STATE HOSPITAL
Danvers, Massachusetts
1878-1992

"The thoughts written on the walls of madhouses by their inmates might be worth publicizing."
~Georg Christoph Lichtenberg

Let's imagine you've just moved into a brand new apartment building. Condominiums, actually. As you walk the wide hallways headed toward your own condo, you hear a sound. Was it a sound *you* made? Or was it something else?

Before you can answer your own question, a dark shadow rushes by you. A rush of cold air raises goose bumps on your arms and the back of your neck.

Will your pace quicken until you reach your apartment door and its relative safety? And will you be safe from whatever is following you, nay *stalking* you, in the hallways?

It could happen.

In fact, it has possibly happened already. In Danvers, Massachusetts, at the Avalon Danvers Apartments, there is a secret past to this trendy new set of condominiums, one that deals in madness, murder, suicide, tragedy, sadness, and abuse.

Before the Avalon Danvers apartment building took shape, the Danvers State Hospital, an institution for the insane that claimed 768 lives, sat on the property. It was an institution so monstrous in size and reputation that it inspired cult fantasy and horror writer H.P. Lovecraft to model the Arkham Sanatorium in his short novel, *The Thing On The Doorstep,* after the Danvers State Hospital, which, in turn, inspired the infamous Arkham Asylum from the *Batman* comic books.

In 1878, the first buildings of the Danvers State Hospital were built and opened for business. Consisting of two center-set administration buildings and two wings to either side for male and female patients, the hospital quickly became recognized for being incredibly self-sufficient. A pond onsite provided water for the buildings, and farms on the property provided work for the patients, as well as food for their consumption. Over the years, a gymnasium, auditorium, and solarium were added to the existing structures, as were an incredibly intricate series of tunnels that ran underneath the asylum. These tunnels, commonplace in nearly every asylum profiled in this book, served the same purposes as the others: discreet patient transfers, employee passageways, storage, and, ultimately, tactful removal of the dead.

Originally, the hospital was designed and built with the maximum population of only 500 patients in mind. But by the mid 1920s, there was said to be well over 2,000 patients interred within the cavernous hospital. Not only were the insane taken in there, but also the drug addicted, alcoholics, homeless, and the destitute. Orphaned children could be found wandering about the hospital as well. Because of the severe overcrowding, drastic measures were taken to quell the more unruly patients. Straight jacketing, chain restraints, various mind-altering drugs, and electroshock therapy were only a few of the actions taken. It is said that the lobotomy was developed and put into use for the first time at Danvers State Hospital as well.

All of these treatments, of course, sparked controversy, and by the 1960s, the inpatient population had begun to dwindle, mostly because of the use of alternative forms of mental health practices that were based around deinstitutionalization and community-based mental health treatments.

In 1992, due to state budget cuts, Danvers was forced to close. It stood empty for thirteen years, rotting and decaying, its ghosts alive within the bricks of their old home. Its most famous moment came in 2001 when filmmakers used the old abandoned asylum for their film *Session 9* starring David Caruso. A tight and atmospheric thriller, *Session 9* used the eerie and often creepy asylum to its best advantage, providing an incredible look at this amazing building from the inside-out in ways that many people have never seen before. However, when filming wrapped, it again stayed empty and rotting. The film did not seem to sway those wanting to demolish the historic old building that had become home to countless spirits of former residents.

In 2004, a private company named Avalon bought Danvers State Hospital and plans were made to demolish a good portion of the outbuildings and wings, while converting the administration wings into condominiums. This was fairly unheard of, mainly due to the fact that the building had already been designated a historic landmark. However, before the hospital was bought by developers, not much interest had been placed in the rehabilitation of the hospital, the demolition of which so many people were now protesting.

Amid these protests, the developers demolished much of the building and its surrounding outbuildings, leaving about one third of the original structure intact.

In April of 2007, while reconstruction was going on, a mysterious fire broke out, consuming four of Avalon Bay's construction trucks as well as four of the apartment complex buildings. The fire was so large and intense that it was visible from Boston, some seventeen miles away. The fire was confined mostly to the buildings under construction on the east end, with only minor scorching on the original spires, due to the excessive heat. A webcam installed by Avalon Bay provided a live feed of the construction process, but at 2:03 a.m. on the night of the fire, the feed cut out and the webcam was disabled. An investigation revealed nothing. There was no evidence to suggest foul play, nor were there any wiring, fuel, or construction issues that pointed toward a reason.

Today, Danvers State Hospital is no more. Nothing is left of the old buildings but the memories of what had once been. The Administration wing, carefully renovated, still hangs on to the look of the old Kirkbride Building.

When the hospital was demolished, did it release the tortured souls of those who had perished there, or did the energy of those poor souls remain, finding shelter in the hallways of a new home?

Before it was demolished, very few paranormal investigators had a chance to investigate Danvers State Hospital. Those who have been lucky enough to investigate, however, reported hearing voices, banging sounds, distant footsteps, and screams. Former employees of Danvers State Hospital also reported the chilling appearance of full-bodied apparitions and of hearing the tortured screams of former patients.

Former employees who have lived on the property have seen full-bodied apparitions of men and women garbed in patient clothes, their eyes cold and blank.

In addition to seeing these ghosts, they also have been visited in their bedrooms. Invisible hands have been known to rip the sheets off of the beds and the tormented screams of the mad would echo throughout the building.

Also, equally troubling, is the fact that during construction, the hospital's old cemetery simply disappeared, only to reappear once more as a series of simple flat stones with numbers upon them ranging from 300 to 600. Were the bodies removed, relocated, and the headstones left in place? Highly doubtful. To this very day, chances are still very good that there are close to 300 bodies still buried on the property.

When the Avalon Danvers Apartments were finally opened, the condos quickly filled up. But the conditions inside met very few expectations. Former residents expressed their disdain for the apartment buildings, saying that the buildings were always cold, the chill unbearable during winter. Plumbing and electrical maintenance was ongoing. It seems as if everything needed to be fixed on a more-than-regular basis. Some residents even complained of hearing footsteps walking up and down the halls at all hours of the night.

It is impossible now to pinpoint exact hotspots inside Danvers State Hospital, mostly because many of those hotspots don't exist anymore. All we have left are the memories of what happened before. But if the statements of the former residents of Avalon Danvers are true, then perhaps a new chapter in paranormal history is being written as I write this.

7.

EASTERN STATE PENITENTIARY
Philadelphia, Pennsylvania
1829-1971

"Prison is no place for anybody to start off at. This is where everybody ends up and they
end up being a loser in life. This is where the ball game begins and only the tough survive."
~California prison offender

It was America's first penitentiary, a place built for the true spiritual redemption of the prisoners who called it home. The initial design concepts were born in Benjamin Franklin's home around 1787, but the official design and construction did not begin until 1821. Completed and opened in 1829, utilizing a revolutionary "wagon wheel" design, Eastern State Penitentiary began in the middle, having a singular tower with seven cell blocks radiating outward, resembling the spokes of a wagon's wheel. This design not only used the space more effectively, it ensured that the guards and administration would be able to oversee all the prisoners easily from one central location.

From the very beginning, the ideas of penitence and redemption played heavily upon the rehabilitation of the prisoners. The warden was required to meet with each prisoner daily and his overseers were required to meet with them three times daily. The cells themselves had small, narrow doorways, requiring prisoners to almost bow before entering their bleak new surroundings. Light came in the form of a thin shaft of sunlight through a single glass skylight, commonly dubbed "The Eye Of God." Within this cell, under the watchful eye of God himself, prisoners would be forced to face the sin and crime they had committed against others.

If they fought their rehabilitation, guards and counselors devised a series of physical and psychological tortures designed to break down the spirit of the condemned. Some were forced outside during winter months and doused with icy water. Others had their tongues chained to their wrists so that they might tear out their own tongue if they struggled. Still others were tossed into "The Hole," a pit dug underneath Cell Block 14 where there was no light, no human contact, and as little food as possible.

And then there was the "Mad Chair," a large barber's chair replete with heavy leather straps situated in its own sealed-off room. The worst of offenders would be strapped into this chair and left alone for days, sealed off from everything. It has been called the Mad Chair for the obvious reasons: men left alone in this chair were said to go mad from being restrained and isolated for so long.

Perhaps the most agonizing part of the rehabilitation process was the fact that each prisoner was, in essence, segregated from his fellow prisoners at all times. Prisoners were not allowed to interact with each other; hoods were forced over their heads whenever they needed to be moved. Time in the exercise yard was limited to two prisoners at a time and high stone walls had been erected around different sections of the yard so that the convicts could not easily communicate with one another. Essentially, Eastern State Penitentiary was one big solitary confinement cell block.

But by 1913, severe overcrowding forced the hands of administrators into eliminating the solitary systems and implementing the now common practice of communal living amongst prisoners. As history has taught us, the implementation of the communal prison isn't without its drawbacks. Murders, rapes, and assaults began to climb amongst the convicts and the guards were obliged to respond, using more force to subdue the violence.

And this was how it was for many years. "Business as usual," as they say. Eastern State Penitentiary was the go-to prison for much of Pennsylvania's convicted criminals, as well as a preferred penitentiary for the worst of America's criminals. In 1929, following his conviction for illegal weapons possession, notorious gangster Al Capone became Eastern State Penitentiary's most famous inmate, staying an agonizingly slow eight months. During this time, it is said that Capone frequently acted out, claiming that he was being haunted by the ghost of a former rival, one he had murdered at the infamous St. Valentine's Day Massacre in Chicago.

In 1945, the only successful escape occurred when bank robber Willie Sutton and eleven other inmates took a year to dig an elaborate ninety-seven-foot-long tunnel that ran underneath the prison wall. This wasn't the only time an escape attempt had been cooked up. During renovations in the 1930s, it is said that thirty incomplete tunnels were uncovered, all bored out by inmates hoping to taste freedom away from Eastern State.

Eastern State Penitentiary was closed in 1971, and many prisoners and guards were transferred to Graterford Prison thirty miles away. In turn, the city of Philadelphia bought up the property with the express intention of redeveloping the land, possibly turning it into a luxury apartment complex surrounded by the old prison walls. But the successful petitioners known as the Eastern State Penitentiary Task Force got Mayor Wilson Goode to halt the proposed redevelopments.

By 1994, Eastern State Penitentiary was open for business once more, this time hosting visitors and tourists interested in the historic value of this former Goliath of prisons. After nearly twenty-five years of emptiness, the old souls of Eastern State Penitentiary were about to meet the new souls.

The reports of paranormal activity began almost immediately, with stories of phantom footsteps in the upper and lower ranges of the cell blocks. Mysterious voices, screams, and taunts could be heard being whispered into the ears of visitors. Apparitions began appearing as shadowy figures inside the decrepit, creepy prison cells. Soon, Eastern State Penitentiary was known not only for its historical significance, but also for its restless spirits still trapped in their cages, still unrepentant, still angry, and some just very, very sad.

Al Capones Cell

Without a doubt, the most famous inmate housed at Eastern State had to be the infamous Chicago Mob kingpin, Alphonse "Al" Capone. Leaving town following the St. Valentine's Day Massacre in 1929 to avoid heat from the cops, Capone and his bodyguard made their way to Philadelphia, where they were picked up for carrying concealed weapons. Sentenced to a year in jail, Capone made the most of his time at Eastern State, living in the lap of luxury. His cell was lavishly decorated, complete with ornate chairs, tasteful paintings, a large cabinet radio, a writing desk, a large opulent rug and deluxe bedding for his large, soft body. He was allowed to make long-distance telephone calls from the warden's office. He was able to meet with anyone he chose, at any time, mostly opting to speak with his lawyers and notorious business associates Frank Nitti, Jack Guzik, and his brother, Ralph.

But all the luxuries in the world weren't enough to calm his nerves. Late into the night, Capone could be heard crying and screaming out, begging to be left alone. But with the exception of Capone himself, the cell remained empty. According to witnesses at the time, Capone claimed that he was being haunted by a spirit named "Jimmy," possibly the ghost of James Clark, one of the men murdered by Capone in the infamous St. Valentine's Day Massacre. Jimmy never appeared to any other prisoner and most thought that Capone was quickly losing what little sanity he had left.

When he left Eastern State later that year, Capone may have been relieved for a time, but his relief did not last. Jimmy's ghost continued to dog Capone's heels until Capone finally hired a well-known psychic named Alice Britt to exorcise Jimmy's enraged spirit. Not long after the séance, it is said that Capone's personal valet, Hymie Cornish, saw the spirit of Jimmy Clark in the lounge area of Capone's apartment. The tall, dark specter stood near the window and stared at Cornish as he dissipated from view. Capone claimed that Jimmy Clark continued to haunt him until his eventual death from syphilis in 1947.

Was Jimmy real? Or was Jimmy merely a figment of Capone's imagination, a manifestation of the guilt he felt for orchestrating the bloodiest mob hit in gangster history? Gangsters of the time were notoriously straight laced, not given to telling tales, and certainly not given to showing weakness through fear or guilt. Whatever Capone was haunted by, he certainly felt it was real.

The Shadow Phantom

The spirit of Jimmy Clark was hardly the only one to haunt Eastern State Penitentiary. The sounds of disembodied screams, loud, echoing footsteps, and the incessant whispers of the dead have been heard throughout the building's seven cell blocks.

But of the seven cell blocks, the ones with seemingly the most activity belong to Cell Blocks 6, 12, and 15. It is in these ranges and walkways that the most paranormal activity occurs. Shadow figures dart and pace about the cells and halls of cell blocks 6 and 12, appearing and disappearing at random. Some have even been known to creep up and down the walls. Usually, the kinetic feelings of being watched accompanies these shadow figures and their appearance is usually met with sheer terror for those lucky enough to catch sight of them.

Several witnesses, independent of one another, have reported the same distinct, yet far-off sounds of laughter, as well as the infamous shadow figures. A locksmith by the name of Gary Johnson, sent to perform some routine restoration work, recalls his own experiences with the ghosts of Cell Block 12.

I had this feeling that I was being watched, but I turned and I'm looking down the block and there's nobody there. A couple of seconds later and I get the same feeling... I'm really being watched! I turn around and I look down the block and shoooom.... this black shadow just leaped across the block!

This shadow figure is one of the most reported in the prison and it always appears in virtually the same way. It is a dark, human-like figure that stands motionless and calm, usually going unnoticed until a visitor or worker gets too close and then it darts away. What it leaves behind are feelings of anger and malevolence, a general feeling of ill will that permeates the conscience of the person he appears to.

It is believed that The Atlantic Paranormal Society (TAPS) captured this Shadow Man during their televised investigation of Eastern State Penitentiary on SyFy Channel's *Ghost Hunters*. It has since become one of the most, if not *the* most, compelling piece of photographic evidence ever collected inside the prison. In grainy night-vision footage, the cloaked specter of a man can be seen running toward the night-vision camera. Then, as if noticing the camera, turns to run back and quickly dissipates into thin air. The apparition was featureless, looking more like the misty vision of a man swathed in a black robe or cape.

Was it a black, misty apparition? Or was it in fact a man in a dark robe?

By their own admission, the TAPS members were out to dinner at the time the apparition was caught on tape in the upper range of Cell Block 12. Is it possible that the apparition was an intruder who sought to hoax a ghost sighting while the building sat empty?

On the other hand, how could a human appear, then disappear so quickly without a trace?

The Haunted Watchtower

Another of Eastern State's more famous spooks is that of the guard who spends his nights within the Watchtower of the prison. His dark figure has been spotted inside the Watchtower, pacing, rifle on his back. Many have assumed that this could be the spirit of a guard who felt such devotion to his job that he still reports to his post each night, or perhaps he bore witness to, or took part in, deeds that have compelled him back to this place. What is certain however, is that his devotion to Eastern State is mirrored by the employees and volunteers of today, those fiercely protective folks who are determined to keep Eastern State Penitentiary the way it is, preserving its heritage for many years to come.

Greta Galuszka, a current employee of Eastern State, pretty much sums up why Eastern State both fascinates and terrifies.

So much did happen here that there's the potential for a lot of unfinished business to be hanging around. And I think that's my fear—to stumble upon some of that unfinished business.

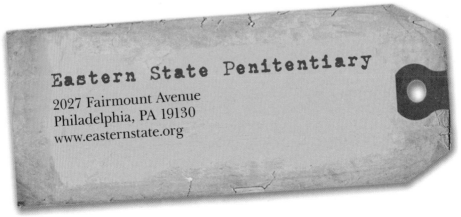

Eastern State Penitentiary
2027 Fairmount Avenue
Philadelphia, PA 19130
www.easternstate.org

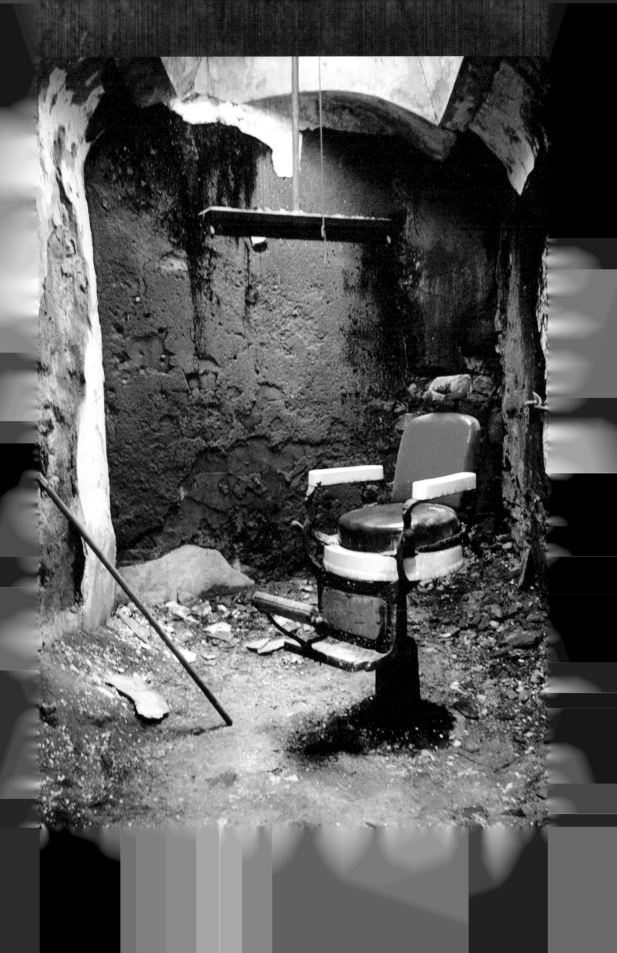

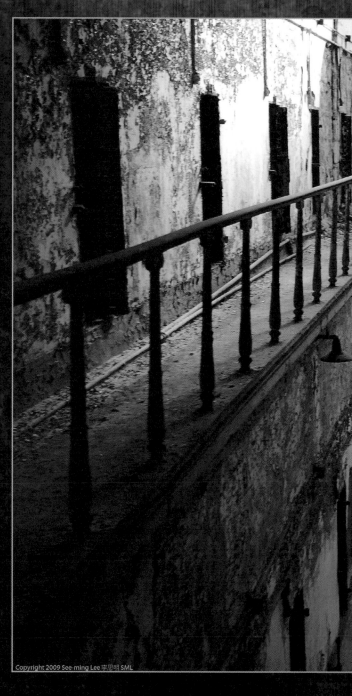

PHOTO: 72 Eastern State Cell Block.
Photo courtesy of See-ming Lee.

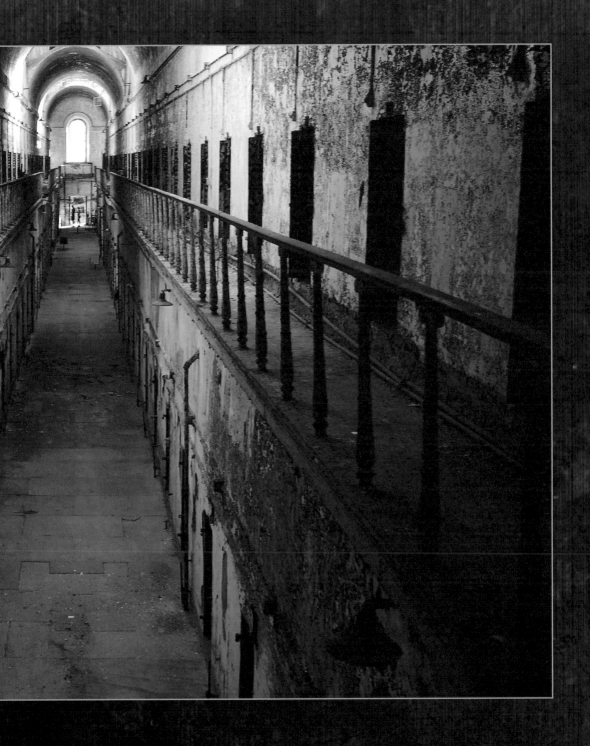

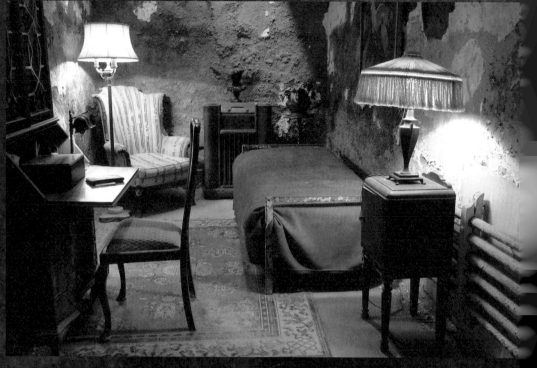

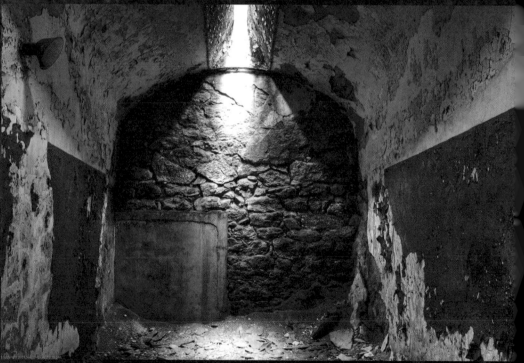

PHOTO: 74 - Eastern State Pen Cell by See-ming Lee
The luxurious cell Capone used for a year, compared to the paltry one enjoyed by the other, less influential prisoners. *Photos courtesy of Adam Jones Ph.D and See-ming Lee.*

8.

PRESTON CASTLE
Ione, California
1894-1960

"Within yourself deliverance must be searched for, because each man makes his own prison."
~Edwin Arnold

It is always sad when a youth goes awry, becoming a criminal statistic, a stigma that will stay wrapped around their necks for the rest of their lives. It is perhaps even sadder when those same criminal children, forgotten by society, become forgotten by God after death claims them. But don't be fooled by the sad tales these young lives tell us now. While they lived, some of these children were well on their way to becoming the next Manson, John Dillinger, or William H. Bonney. They may have aspired to those heights or that may have been the only option for a life. For those children abandoned by society and adopting a criminal lifestyle to survive, the Preston School of Industry was built and dedicated. Because of its stately Romanesque architecture, locals began referring to it as Preston Castle, a nickname that has stuck and become more popular than the official name.

Built between 1890 and 1894, Preston Castle opened proudly as a detention center for wayward youths, boys who had run afoul of the law. The bricks that make up its thick walls were cut and shipped by the inmates of California's San Quentin and Folsom Prisons, two infamous penitentiaries known almost exclusively for their brutal population. With four stories, a basement, and a soaring bell tower, Preston Castle owns the hill it sits atop, dominating the skyline view and all 230 acres it sprawls across.

Boys of every age and of every background were brought here for a variety of offenses, ranging from simple pick-pocketing to burglary and murder. A few of the more famous inmates included actor Rory Calhoun, country singer Merle Haggard, Jack Benny's sidekick, Eddie Anderson, and tennis great Pancho Gonzales. They were prisoners, but the faculty treated them more as students and attempted to show them different paths they could take.

Because of their wayward and antisocial behaviors, they were taught trades that could be used in everyday life when they were returned to the streets. This is why, officially, Preston Castle is known as Preston School of Industry. Virtually every trade imaginable was taught at the school, such as metal working, farming, and tailoring. There was a bakery, wood shop, and metal shop on the school grounds. Even the art of butchering cattle and swine was taught (a lucrative trade, yet still disturbing to imagine children engaging in the act).

Although the staff treated the boys like students, it was the guards who treated them like inmates, doling out harsh punishments and abuse for even the slightest offenses. Infraction cards were handed out regularly for everything from smoking to trying to escape. It has been speculated that the guards saw the boys for what they truly were: stone-cold killers and criminals. In fact, many former employees of Preston Castle can attest to the fact that these boys, young as they were, were just as cold and dangerous as the men incarcerated at Corcoran, San Quentin, or Folsom prisons.

The Murder of Anna Corbin

In February of 1950, Anna Corbin, a 52-year-old woman who served as the Castle's head housekeeper, was found brutally murdered in a closet near the basement kitchen. She had been viciously beaten and strangled, the hemp cord still wrapped around her neck, her body rolled up into a carpet. It was staff member Lillian McDowell who discovered Anna locked in the closet. Because the door had been locked, not only were students investigated, but key-carrying staff members as well. In all, 657 wards and all of the staff were interrogated by presiding Superintendent Robert A. Chandler. But true suspicion only fell on one man.

So how did a kind and pretty 52-year-old woman end up at a reform school in Ione, California? Born January 16, 1898, in Kansas, as Anna Laura Lawton, she eventually married a local truck driver name Robert Corbin sometime in 1918, birthing son Harold a year later. They had moved to Colorado, and, eventually, to a town called Whittier in East Los Angeles, California. By 1930, Anna and Robert had daughter, Avis. When World War II broke out in 1941, both Robert and his son, Harold, were drafted to fight. Two years later, Anna's heart would be broken when she learned that her son had been killed in action. His grave still sits in the Golden Gate National Cemetery in San Bruno, California. Anna's husband returned home in 1945, following the surrender of Japan, but died two years later in 1947 in Napa, California.

A widowed mother with a 17-year-old daughter, Anna soon found herself in dire straits with no prospects for the future. On the cusp of the 1950s, Anna would have been forced to take any job imaginable in order to support her daughter. While still grieving her son and husband, Anna now found herself as a housekeeper to 657 wayward youths who desperately needed a mother in their lives as much as Anna needed to be a mother.

But not everyone found comfort with Anna. On February 23, 1950, staff member Lillian McDowell discovered the body of Anna Corbin stuffed in a rolled up carpet in the far corner of the basement. She had been bludgeoned repeatedly and a rope was found wrapped around her neck. When the wards of Preston Castle found out that their beloved, motherly Anna had been murdered, several were reported to have said that if the assailant were another ward of the Castle, retribution would be doled out swiftly and violently. In the end, after the list of suspects had been exhausted, only one name remained as an air-tight suspect.

A 19 year-old black man named Eugene Monroe was arrested for the murder, based on eyewitness testimony placing him outside Corbin's office around the time of its occurrence. Further inquiry revealed that he had been in trouble for burglary elsewhere in the state of California, probably bringing him to Preston Castle until his 21st birthday, when he would face release onto an unsuspecting world. Blood was found on Eugene's belt, and inmate James Mercer testified that he had seen Eugene Monroe burning his clothes in the building's incinerator. Prior to his incarceration, he had been suspected of murdering a 17-year-old girl in Los Angeles, California.

Monroe was tried three times for the murder of Anna Corbin, with two of the trials ending in hung juries. Yet, at the third trial, Monroe was acquitted of the crime due to a lack of physical evidence linking him to Anna's death. A year later, Monroe was arrested again, this time in Tulsa, for the rape and murder of a woman similar in age to Anna Corbin. He never admitted fault in Anna's murder and many believe that it wasn't him at all. With a building so full of troubled boys and young men, it is something of a miracle that no other murders occurred.

Anna was especially well liked amongst the staff and the inmates, making her murder all that much more intriguing. Her pretty smile and comforting disposition was said to have had a very calming influence over boys in her charge.

Today, investigators and employees often report the sounds of a woman screaming in the distance, the sound reverberating throughout the empty stone halls, and eerie white mists have been seen around the area where Anna's body was found. Most compelling, though, are the gifts of flowers that visitors leave in Anna's apartment. An offering of flowers in memory of Anna seems to bring the spirit out, revealing herself on EVPs and in the warm feeling of her presence near you. Paranormal researchers have tried to communicate with Anna in the past, but her EVPs are notoriously tight lipped about her murderer's identity.

However, she does not seem to be bound by the tragedy of her past life. It is possible that today she presides over the spirits of boys who cannot pass onto the next world, making sure they are not alone, that they are warm and well cared for.

The Ghosts of Samuel Goins and Joe Lopez

Violence was not uncommon amongst the boys, but deaths *because* of violence were. Boys would scrap with each other, settle their arguments with fists, as was common for boys of their predicament. In all, the Preston Castle graveyard holds only twenty-three gravestones. Seventeen of them were victims of tuberculosis and typhoid fever.

Only one boy, 20-year-old Samuel Goins, died unnaturally at the end of a gun. He had been shot and killed by a guard as he and fellow inmate Joe Lopez tried to make an escape from the school just two months before his release date. At the time, and even in retrospect, the escape attempt and subsequent shooting seemed a tad suspect. But make no mistake, Goins was at Preston Castle for a reason: he was a convicted burglar with a fiery temperament. His partner in crime, Joe Lopez, died eight months later under mysterious circumstances.

Whatever the facts may be behind Samuel's and Joe's deaths, what *is* clear is that their spirits still walk the halls of Preston Castle. Footsteps have been heard in nearly every part of the school and the voices of young boys come from out of nowhere during EVP sessions.

There is also said to be two dark wraiths that wander the halls of Preston Castle, anger boiling up when new souls arrive in search of spirits. Most investigators theorize that Goins and Lopez are the dark ghosts that Anna Corbin's spirit repeatedly tries to warn the innocent about. Together, they push, scratch, and pinch those innocent bystanders who come looking for them.

Even in death, these two partners in crime work together to terrorize and violate as many people as they can. One can imagine that they enjoy what they do, especially now that they have no bodies to hold their anger and psychotic behavior at bay.

The ghostly events at Preston Castle are, admittedly, not as plentiful as, say, the Ohio State Reformatory or Trans-Allegheny Lunatic Asylum. But not all ghostly encounters need to be terrifying in order to be considered valid. Preston Castle was a place of healing, like Waverly Hills, where lives were turned around and the souls of children were saved before it was too late. The murder of Anna Corbin, and the vengeful spirits of Joe Lopez and Samuel Goins, as horrible as their stories are, all seem to reinforce the idea that in death, as in life, there is a sense of good and evil that continually fights against one another.

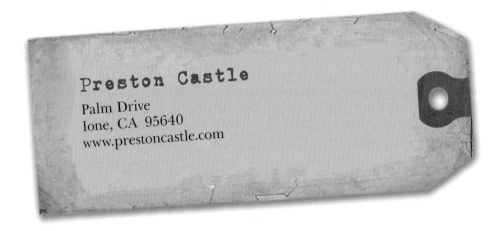

Preston Castle

Palm Drive
Ione, CA 95640
www.prestoncastle.com

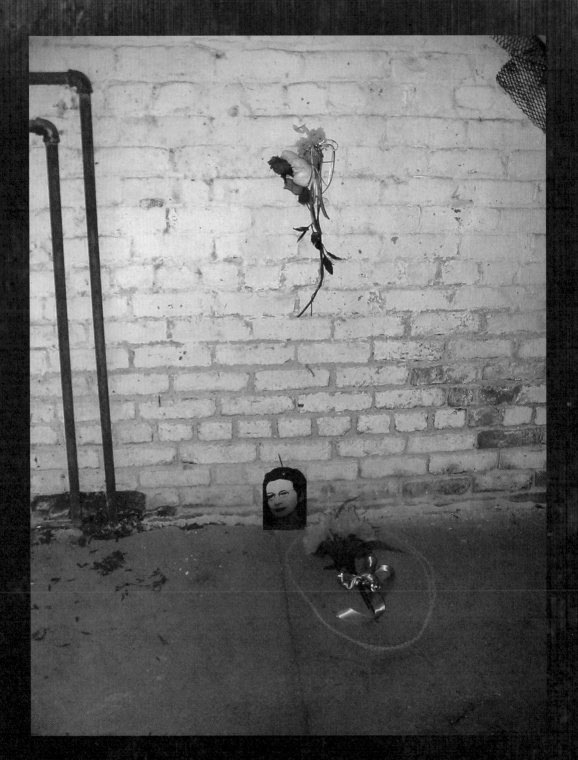

PHOTO: 46-PRESTON CASTLE ANNA CORBIN SHRINE
The basement room where Anna's body was found is a favorite stop for those wishing to pay tribute to her by leaving offerings of flowers and cards. *Photo courtesy of Mattie Parfitt.*

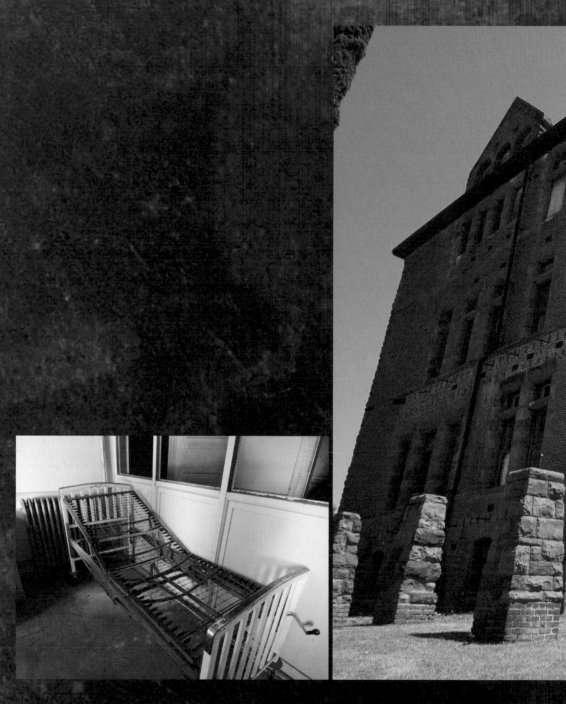

The infirmary at Preston Castle, one of the more common places where Joe Lopez and Samuel Goins—among others—are said to haunt. *Photo courtesy of Lori Mattas.*

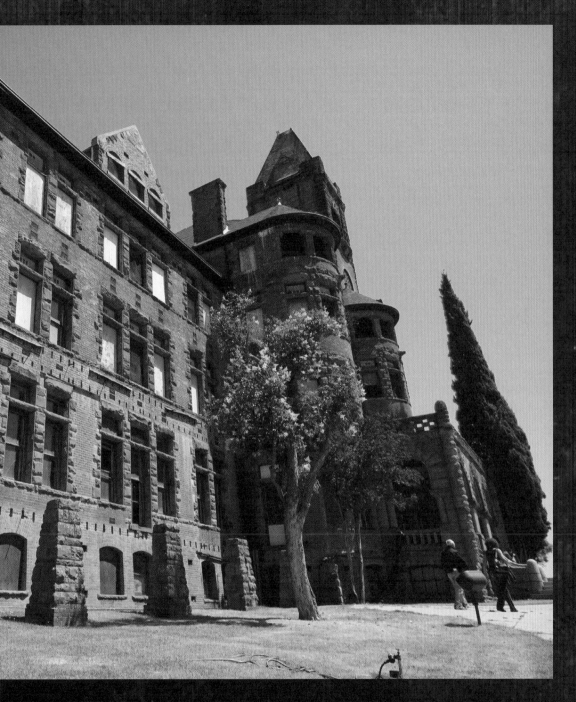

PHOTO: 82 – PRESTON LoriMattas 0185

The Preston School of Industry, aka Preston Castle. *Photo courtesy of Lori Mattas.*

9.

THE ASYLUMS OF ILLINOIS

"What is the most innocent place in any country? Is it not the insane asylum? These people drift through life truly innocent, unable to see into themselves at all."

~Arthur Miller

Ashmore Estates
Ashmore, Illinois

Located out in the middle of rural Ashmore, Illinois, lies a brick building that many consider to be one of the most haunted in the state. Ashmore Estates has long been considered a haunted building, but has been off limits for the better part of twenty years since its closing. It stands out like a sore thumb, a gigantic brick Goliath of a building surrounded by cornfields. Desolate and unforgiving, Ashmore Estates stands starkly against the horizon and almost screams at you to be afraid.

Surprisingly, most people improperly regard Ashmore Estates as a former insane asylum; it actually began in 1857 as part of the Coles County Almshouse, housing homeless families, vagrants, and orphans. Over its forty-year history as a poorhouse, the Coles County Almshouse buried almost 200 residents. But it was a place that seemed to do more good than bad. Nancy Andrews Swinford, a former tenant of the poorhouse and daughter of Almshouse superintendent Leo Roy Andrews, told the *Times-Courier*:

> They were warm and had good food on the table. And, they loved working and earning their keep. They weren't moochers.... They mostly grew their own food, did their own butchering, and smoked the meat. They smoked their own bacon and hams in the smoke house, they killed and dressed all their own chickens, and made their own butter.

Closing its doors to the poor of Coles County in 1956, it was purchased by Ashmore Estates, Inc. and reopened as a home for mentally impaired men, women, and children. Ashmore Estates, at that time, essentially acted as a substitute hospital for the massive overflows of patients at the larger, not quite as scary, state hospital.

Floors one and two housed the mentally retarded, the depressed, and the only slightly deranged. Floor three, however, housed the more dangerous, more hostile patients. It has been said that some of those patients came to Ashmore Estates possessed of demons. When the patients died, the demons remained behind, multiplying and exploiting the fractured minds of the residents.

Ashmore Estates, as a hospital, remained in use until 1987, when a severe lack of funding forced it to close. In that time, it is believed that over a hundred people died there, their bodies buried in the Ashmore Estates cemetery.

In 2006, it came into private ownership and was opened to paranormal groups for investigations, as well as to the paying public for haunted tours. Almost immediately, word got out that there was some heavy paranormal activity going on behind the heavy wooden doors of Ashmore Estates. Physical attacks, whispering voices, and full-bodied apparitions have been experienced on a regular basis, and many people experience what investigators classify as possession. In one fairly famous event, a meteorologist doing a live internet broadcast for a local TV station was apparently picked up and thrown to the ground.

Joseph Oliver Bloxom, a resident of the poor farm whose life ended when he was sideswiped by a train, continues to walk the halls of Ashmore, a place he considered the only true home he had ever known. He sometimes appears in darkened corridors as a shadowy apparition and when paranormal investigators capture EVPs of a male voice, it is generally accredited to Joe Bloxom.

Elva Skinner, a pretty little girl who was about 9 at the time of her death, met her fate in a horrific fire that broke out in Ashmore Estates in February 1880. EVPs of her tiny, heart-wrenching voice have been captured pleading for help and begging for her "mama." Her sad spirit wanders the halls of the second and third floor, appearing in the decrepit hallways and in the dirty and broken windows of the upper floors, still looking for her mother, still looking for help.

Bartonville State Hospital
Peoria, Illinois

In the early years of the 20th century, a mute by the name of Bookbinder was admitted to the mental hospital in Bartonville, Illinois. A strong, but somewhat disturbed man, Old Book (as he came to be known) was given the task of digging graves for the dead in Bartonville State Hospital's patient graveyards. He attended and wept at each funeral, at first mystifying the staff. After all, the deceased was almost always a stranger and rarely known to anyone. Yet Old Book still found himself clutching the old Elm tree in the cemetery, weeping madly for the man or woman he was about to help return to the Earth.

For years, he afforded the same courtesy to everyone who arrived at his four graveyards, until one day, sadly, it was Old Book's turn to pass on. Dr. George Zeller, the head physician of Bartonville State Hospital, would preside over the service in the same way he had presided over all the other funerals. Because he was so well liked and showed so much respect for the dead patients in the past, almost 300 people, including some patients, nurses, and doctors showed up to pay their respects to Old Book.

Just as the choir finished the last lines of "Rock of Ages," the pallbearers grasped the ropes suspending Old Book's coffin over the open grave, stooped forward, and with a powerful effort began to lift the coffin so that the crossbeams could be removed and the coffin could be gently lowered into the grave. By the count of three, they pulled heavily on the ropes and almost instantly found themselves lying flat on their backs. The coffin offered no resistance and bounced into the air as if it were empty. At that time, everyone heard the familiar wails of Old Book near the graveyard Elm tree that he always frequented, sobbing loudly.

Shocked and curious to see if Old Book truly was dead or not, a few of the pallbearers stepped forward to open the coffin. The weeping stopped. Old Book was inside, dead, and no longer visible at the graveyard Elm. Over the years, people have attempted to cut down the tree and have even tried to burn it. But once they start, they are shocked and frightened by the sound of horrific wailing emanating from the tree. It was decided to leave the tree as a marker for the otherwise unmarked grave of Bartonville's most beloved patient, Old Book.

Pretty good story, eh? Indeed, and a chilling one at that, especially since it really happened. Don't believe me? You could have asked the 300 other people who saw it and they would back up the man testifying to what happened that day in the graveyard, Dr. George Zeller. In his autobiography, *Befriending The Bereft*, Dr. Zeller told the story of Old Book and many other strange occurrences that happened at the Bartonville State Hospital. Dr. Zeller believed it when it happened to him and he has the eyewitnesses to back it up.

Bartonville State Hospital's sad life began in 1887, when it first opened to receive patients, its façade an imposing, medieval castle-like design. But by 1897, the hospital lay in ruins, demolished. Seems that when Bartonville State was being built, they situated it over a series of old abandoned mines. As the mines slowly began to collapse, the foundation began to crumble. Reopened and stronger than ever, in 1902, under the direction of Dr. George Zeller, Bartonville instituted a revolutionary mental health design that precluded bars on the windows and instituted a series of thirty-three cottages for the patients to reside in instead of dormitory-style wings and blocks. Bartonville State Hospital also boasted a home for the nurses, a chapel, its own bakery, laundry, and power station.

Like many hospitals of its time, Bartonville quickly became known as home for many of the patients, most of whom resided there all their lives. Over the seventy years Bartonville State Hospital was in business, the hospital saw enough deaths to fill four graveyards, including the one Old Book and his beloved Elm tree are said to inhabit.

When it closed in 1972, and came under private ownership in 1980, amateur ghost hunters and vandals soon discovered just how haunted Bartonville State Hospital really was: full-bodied apparitions, the sounds of screams and whispers in your ears. Doors would open and close on their own, and the tell-tale sound of footsteps, a haunted house specialty, have also been heard.

Alas, most of the older buildings and cottages have been demolished, but the main building and the graveyards still remain. Rumor has it that they are planning to use it as office space. Bartonville, like many of the other hospitals in this book, is a vortex of pain and suffering, but also promises a glimmer of hope to those seeking healing.

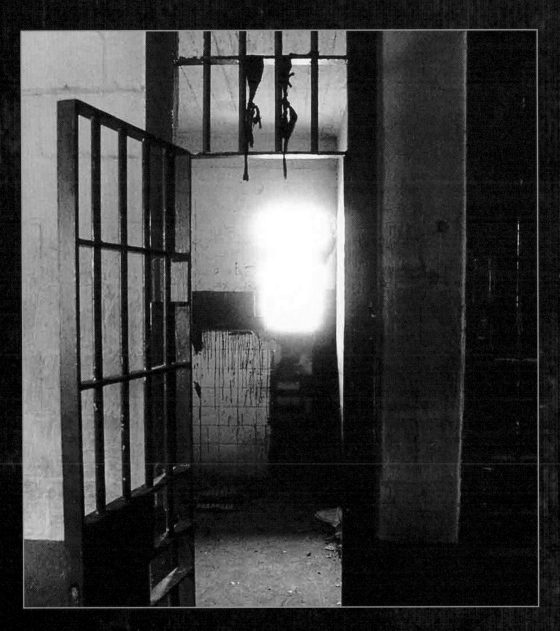

PHOTO: 15 - ASYLUM DOOR

10.

WYOMING FRONTIER PRISON
Rawlins, Wyoming
1872-1997

"In prison, those things withheld from and denied to the prisoner become precisely what he wants most of all."

~Eldridge Cleaver

When the first cornerstone of the Wyoming Frontier Prison was laid in 1888, few realized that it would be another thirteen years before the prison would be accepting its first prisoners. Quite a long time to be under construction, but funding issues and the notoriously schizophrenic weather of Wyoming hampered the fledgling prison until its opening in 1901.

With no electricity or running water, Wyoming Frontier Prison held a whopping 104 cells that housed over 13,000 inmates during its entire 80-year run. Additional cell blocks were added over the years in an effort to curtail the growing population of the West's most lawless men. In addition to the cold and dank cells, the prison came equipped with a torturous dungeon, several different types of solitary confinement cells, and a whipping post that saw more than its share of disciplinary cases reduced to bloody heaps of crying men.

The prison's Death Row didn't come until the mid 1930s. Up until then, a type of traveling gallows was employed and dispatched to different counties and cities in need of such equipment. The original gallows scaffold that sits at the prison today is the same one that took the life of lawman-turned-murderer Tom Horn in 1903.

After eighty years of housing the West's most lethal and notorious murderers, rustlers, and thieves, the Wyoming Frontier Prison closed its doors in 1981. But eighty years of murder, mayhem, and general anarchy left its mark on the prison. Oppressive conditions and intolerable cruelties committed against the inmates by guards and fellow convicts alone resulted in the deaths of hundreds of people. Like most prisons, negative energy is abundant here and it doesn't dissipate over time. It only grows and grows, and the ghostly manifestations that continue to plague the prison are testimony to that theory.

Two inmates in the dungeon died from the extreme cold within the solitary confinement areas, which prompted the administration to stop using those cells until a better heating system could be implemented. Because this was the place where the more mentally unhinged prisoners were taken when acting out, it is very probable that the horror of their disease left its mark on the walls and creates a thick atmosphere within.

A guard committed suicide in one of the guard towers, succumbing to the immense pressure of the stress from working there. The Death House saw the executions of fourteen people over its lifetime. A number of inmates were killed while trying to escape, and the number of murders committed by inmates on other inmates was incredibly high. All of these things create an atmosphere of hostility, danger, and incredibly charged negative energy.

In each of the cell blocks, shadowy apparitions of the prison's dead have been spotted, walking about unfazed by the living, as they go about their business. This is generally referred to as a Residual Haunting. As noted earlier, a Residual Haunting is the so-called playback of a past event. The apparitions involved are not so much spirits or ghosts, but are more like video recordings of an event that took place sometime in the past. It may be a mundane or mediocre event, but it was significant enough to imprint itself on the fabric of time. By comparison, an Intelligent Haunting is when the spirit wants you to notice it and will respond to your questions, commands, or emotional state in an attempt to communicate. This type of haunting occurs at the Wyoming penitentiary as well, coming in the forms of knockings, bangings, and EVPs that answer specific questions with pertinent answers.

Disembodied voices, sounds of cell doors banging shut, and the eerie knocking of boot heels on the stone floors have all been reported. In nearly every case, the sounds have been preceded by the creepy feeling of being watched by unseen eyes. EVPs have captured aggressive voices, threatening harm to anyone who attempts to enter the dungeons. Being that many of the inmates who ended up there were mentally unbalanced, it is no surprise that people sometimes come into contact with a crazed spirit wishing them harm.

The Ghost of Andrew Pixley

One spirit in particular at the prison is said to be that of Andrew Armandoz Benavidez, more commonly known as Andrew Pixley. He was a man of Native American descent who had once served in the Army to avoid jail time for passing bad checks. His life was spent wandering from one petty crime to another. But his life changed drastically, as did the lives of an entire family, on August 7, 1964. He was admittedly quite drunk when he stumbled upon the Wort Motor Hotel in Jackson, Wyoming.

Illinois Circuit Judge Robert McAuliffe and his family had been in the midst of a five-week road trip, vacationing across the country and staying in at-the-time luxurious motor inns. Leaving their three young daughters to sleep in the hotel room, Judge McAuliffe and his wife attended a show at a theater inside the hotel.

Little is known as to what possessed Andrew Pixley that night. In later statements, he claims to not remember a thing—that because he was an Indian, he "couldn't do that." But whatever thoughts had been swirling about his brain, they now compelled him to remove the screen from a window in the rear and climb into a room, where he found 12 and 8-year-old Debby and Cindy McAuliffe asleep.

The shrieks of terror from their daughters and the horrendous sound of a struggle brought Debby and Cindy's parents running and they were horrified to find a strange man, wearing no shirt or shoes, passed out on the floor of their motel room, the lifeless bodies of Debby and Cindy lying nearby. Debby had been bludgeoned with a rock, Cindy had been strangled. Both girls had been raped. Their third daughter, 6-year-old Susan, had been untouched and unharmed. When police finally arrived, they found Judge McAuliffe holding Pixley down to the floor as he wept, "My God! This man has killed my babies!"

Pixley claimed he remembered nothing, but under the influence of hospital-administered sodium pentothal, he made a statement to police that was withheld from the media and the public until after the coming trial. Pixley said he remembered drinking earlier that evening, but could not remember killing the girls—Pixley also remembered drinking with another man earlier that same evening, but that his mind had drawn a blank since he'd last seen that person.

Dr. William Karn, Jr. of the Wyoming State Hospital examined Pixley and found him to be of sound mind, but that he was most definitely an "incurable sociopath." When pressed to offer an idea as to whether or not Pixley had killed the girls as they slept, Karn replied, "It meant a lot more to Pixley to kill the girls while they were awake." Hearing this brutally honest and chilling affirmation of Pixley's demented persona, Judge McAuliffe rose from his seat and rushed at Pixley before he was restrained by the bailiffs on duty.

Because of the brutality of the crime, citizens of Jackson quickly began to rail against Pixley, forcing officials to move him from the city and into a different jail for his own safety. Lynch mob justice, while antiquated, was still a prevalent fear in the old cowboy town of Jackson. In time, while Pixley maintained that he remembered nothing of the murders and uttered a laugh witnesses describe as "creepy" when he was sentenced to death, his sentence was carried out in 1965 at Wyoming's gas chamber at the Frontier Prison. After the execution, while guards were cleaning out Pixley's cell, they found a crude etching he had made of two very familiar young girls in the paint of his cell wall.

Pixley was a violent man who made life difficult for the guards and other inmates while he awaited his execution. In life, he was a violent, aggressive man.

This did not change when Pixley was executed.

He became a violent, aggressive spirit, wandering the Death House where he spent his last days, tormenting the living as he had in life. Visitors have described being grabbed, pushed, and scratched, presumably by the larger-than-life ghost of Andrew Pixley, but in a prison so full of negative energy, the bearer of the aggression could be anyone. That still doesn't stop paranormal groups from trying to reach out to the unrepentant killer.

Different paranormal groups who have investigated the Death House at the Frontier Prison recall feeling uneasy and afraid while in the Death House. Recently, the Cheyenne Paranormal Investigations team explored the prison, conducting EVP sessions in an effort to get a hold of the violent ghost of Andrew Pixley.

During the EVP session, Tomlinson asked the ghost of Pixley, "Do you know how you died?"

The answer came later when she reviewed the data on her digital recorder. What investigator Stacie Tomlinson received still gives her nightmares. Immediately following her question, the faint, bloodcurdling scream of a child wailing "Noooo!" could be heard in the distance, something that definitely wasn't heard at the original session.

Was it the sound of Debby or Cindy's cries of terror as Andrew Pixley had his way with them, frozen in time for all eternity? Like all paranormal evidence, it is always open to interpretation. But it still manages to chill the blood and send shivers that last for years, doesn't it? Even if the investigators hadn't known the tragedy behind the McAuliffe murders, the mere presence of such a scream would be enough to have people swearing off the prison for decades.

Sometime after the murders of their children, Judge Robert McAuliffe and his wife, Betty, divorced. He remarried, had a son, and died April 1, 1998 of a heart attack. His former wife passed on in 2010, still referring to herself as the wife of

Judge Robert McAuliffe. Their surviving daughter, Susan, is now married and has five children of her own. Life has gone on for the McAuliffe family and the wounds of the past may have healed.

But for Andrew Pixley, he is a permanent fixture in what can only be described as Hell on Earth: forever imprisoned, forever damned with the screams of his victims tormenting his every second.

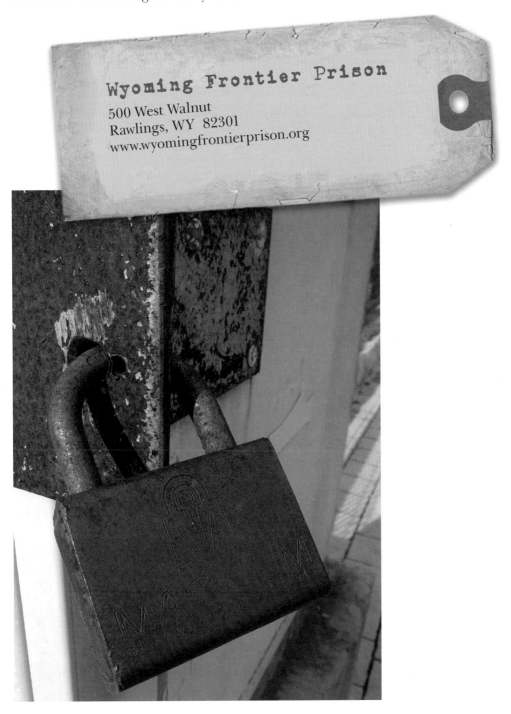

Wyoming Frontier Prison

500 West Walnut
Rawlings, WY 82301
www.wyomingfrontierprison.org

PHOTO 5 OLD RUSTY LOCK

11.

CENTRAL STATE HOSPITAL
Indianapolis, Indiana
1848-1994

"Mental illness is nothing to be ashamed of, but stigma and bias shame us all."

~Bill Clinton

Like many of the hospitals for the insane, Central State Mental Institution, again, is fairly common. Not much distinguishes it from the more notorious hospitals, but what makes Central State so special is the fact that it is just as haunted, if not more, than those other more infamous hospitals. It is also one that barely anyone is aware of outside of the city of Indianapolis. But ask any citizen of the downtown area about Central State Mental Institution and they will tell you that it is one of the most haunted places in the State of Indiana.

Opened in 1848 as the Indiana Hospital for the Insane, its staff of doctors cared for only five patients in a single building. But by the time 1928 rolled around, the population had ballooned to a massive 3,000 patients and the number of buildings had expanded to include wards for the criminally insane, hospital wards to treat the physically ill, an occupational therapy work farm, a bakery, firehouse, cannery, bowling alley, and an amusement hall—all manned by patients under the guidance of mentors and doctors. It was a city unto itself that barely needed the interaction of the outside world to survive. Likely, it was the outside world that had helped to mold the troubled souls within.

Luckily, Central State did not stay overcrowded for long. By the mid 1930s, hospitals in Logansport, Madison, and Richmond relieved the burden of over-crowding from Central State, and the hospital began to serve only those 38 counties within the immediate area.

Sadly, what became of Pennhurst, Danvers, and Weston also affected Central State.

First, massive budget cuts forced the termination of many employees and groundskeepers. As a result, many of the buildings on the campus became un-sound due to the lack of upkeep. By the late 1970s, many of the buildings had to be razed because they were in such poor condition and lacked proper mainte-nance. Grass grew higher, weeds began to invade the once pristine lawns, and the overgrowth of trees and shrubs began to overshadow the buildings themselves.

Second, the ever darkening cloud of patient abuse began to surface as allega-tions began to accumulate regarding the nurses, attendants, and orderlies and their treatment of the patients. Early in the hospital's history, the more violent, criminally insane patients were housed underground in the vast network of tunnels and cells in the basement areas. They were left there in chains, shackled to the walls, as doctors and nurses practiced "retraining exercises," drastic forms of therapy that attempted to reverse whatever mental illness the patient was suffering. After these practices were made public in 1894, the use of restraints was limited to the patients most prone to violent, physical outbursts. Central State tried to make an effort to remain on the positive side of rehabilitation until its closing in 1994. The abuses, it has been said, occurred due mainly to understaffing and poor training. Medical attendants, not doctors, were left in charge of patients much of the time and the long hours, trifling pay, and hazardous work conditions brought the worst out of the attendants.

But let's not let them off the hook just yet.

It was widely reported that, in addition to the incarceration of the more violent inmates being shackled in the basement, those in the so-called "normal" wards were forced to sleep on piles of straw under leaking roofs. Those fortunate enough to have a bed were strapped into them for hours, sometimes days at a time. Even the window wells were used to restrain patients: bars across the window wells turned them into small cages and ensured that the patients could be outside in the sunlight, but restricted from walking about freely. Attendants were known to frequently strike their patients, punish them for talking to other patients, withhold food rations, and lock them in closets.

Over time, though, reforms began to sweep across the nation and a more humane route of dealing with mental illness was implemented. Treatment, rather than restraint, became the norm, and in time, Central State regained its reputation, following a strict code of compassionate conduct that superintendents insisted upon.

But it was a new rash of patient abuse allegations that finally closed the doors of Central State Mental Hospital for good. Perhaps the abuse and neglect never truly ended; indeed, it is possible that the abuse continued, unabated, for years. Whatever the case may have been, the abuses came to an end in 1994 with the incredibly public investigation into the deaths of two of their patients. Housed in the Bahr Building, a ward generally reserved for the more violent patients, June Christy Highsaw and Lydia Shelby both died in 1991 from different forms of patient abuse. Another patient, Linda Heine, had died while taking a bath in 1992, though no evidence of drowning was found. All three were volatile schizophrenics and all were housed in the same building under the same staff.

June Highsaw first entered Central State Hospital in 1970 as a 14-year-old girl suffering from paranoid schizophrenia and mild mental retardation. June had endured a vicious sexual assault at the hospital and had become pregnant by her attacker. Doctors at the hospital had performed an abortion on Highsaw sometime later that left her just as traumatized as her initial attack.

On November 4th of 1991, she suffered and died from hypothermia after she had been allowed to sleep in her own room while two windows remained open, allowing subzero temperatures to waft in from the outside. The coroner's report stated that she had massive amounts of psychiatric drugs in her system, making her body unable to regulate her body temperature. At the time of her death, orderlies and nurses were either napping or playing cards when they were supposed to be looking after her.

Lydia, like June Highsaw, suffered from paranoid schizophrenia and mental retardation; it is possible that violent outbursts led to a glut of psychotropic drugs being administered into her system, which led to acute cardiac arrest. While an internal investigation into the matter revealed no blame or wrongdoings, Governor Evan Bayh ordered a full, state-run investigation into the practices at Central State. Head nurse Ruth Stanley resigned over the allegations of neglect, abuse, and racial discrimination, even though the courts eventually cleared the staff of any wrong doing, indicting five attendants and orderlies for everything from theft to rape and sexual battery.

Purchased by the city of Indianapolis in 2003, the campus of the old Central State Mental Hospital now houses a fire station, a stable for the Metropolitan Mounted Police of Indianapolis, and a museum documenting the history of medicine in Indiana. There are even playgrounds, soccer and softball fields where old dormitories used to sit. Eventually, many of the buildings at the center of the asylum, dubbed "The Seven Steeples" because there were seven wings, each with its own tower, were demolished, leaving only the Administration Building. Some say the trapped energy from the Seven Steeples congregated in the Administration Building after their destruction. Psychics have claimed that an energy vortex swirls inside, like a tornado of energy attracting and feeding the souls of those still trapped there.

And, of course, there are the stories. Stories that began almost as soon as the doors closed for good. Stories that make Indianapolis drivers speed up as they pass the old Central State Hospital grounds. Administration workers, groundskeepers, and even the residents of surrounding homes all tell different, chilling tales of haunted souls, of screams in the night, and of restless spirits still wandering the hospital grounds, even now looking for a way back home.

The Hospital Grounds

The grounds themselves are eerily quiet, and as soon as you enter through the gates and pass by the old security checkpoint booth, it tends to feel as if an overwhelming cloud of gloom falls over you. Structures like the Bolton and Evans Buildings to the right are silent, their broken windows, graffittied walls, and bolted doors a stark contrast to the soccer fields and playgrounds that lie just over 400 feet away. The Bahr Building, home to the criminally insane, sits to the left and is separated by an immense amount of foliage and trees. One can barely make out the building until you walk right up to it. Of all of the buildings still standing at Central State, it is the Bahr Building that seemed to fill me with the most dread. It gave off an aura of tension that resulted in a primordial fear of the unknown. Had the door not been bolted shut, I would have delighted in testing the boundaries the spirits of the Bahr Building had put up.

Travel up the path a ways and you will find the Administration and Power Station Buildings. The feeling of being watched only intensifies as you get closer to these buildings and it is not from the glare of policemen who patrol the grounds vigilantly. These stares come from inside, looking out upon the day. You can feel them upon you.

Having visited the abandoned hospital for myself, I now have no doubt that many of the stories you will hear in this chapter could have actually happened. Central State teems with a spiritual energy that I had not yet felt before and it was exhilarating.

In fact, while I was walking around the perimeter of the old Men's Recreation and Carpentry Buildings, I actually heard the fleeting voices of two men speaking as I went back to my truck. I had parked only a matter of ten feet away from the buildings, but the voices were so loud and so close to me that I thought that one of the policemen had walked up behind me to oust me from the property. When I turned, I saw nothing. Of the two voices, I only understood one of them. He had said, "What are you doing here?" Not only was I completely alone when I heard the voices, but I had just finished peering into some old windows of the Carpentry Building, reveling in the majestic decay and solitude of the structure. Had anyone human said anything to me, I would have heard *and* seen them. I tell you, it was that close.

I wished then that I had picked up my digital voice recorder instead of my camera. It still gives me chills when I think about it.

Because the hospital is nestled in a central part of the inner city of Indianapolis, many drivers and casual observers have reported scores of chilling sights as they have passed by, seeing the apparitions of patients clad only in their hospital gowns, wandering about the lawns behind the big black iron fence. One spirit, who should be commended for his eternal optimism, has been seen on numerous occasions by neighbors, passersby, and ground workers alike. He runs from the hospital, clad in his gown, toward the gates. As his spirit finally touches freedom on neighboring Washington Street, he simply vanishes into thin air. Obviously, one would think of this as some sort of residual energy playing over and over again like a tape recorder stuck on play, but without further investigation, one can't help but wonder.

One area of the campus that drew the attention of night watchmen more than any other was Central State's famous "Grove of Trees." Within this thoroughly spooky thicket of tall, flowing trees are the quick, blur-like forms of shadow people and the plaintive wailing of crying and screaming. Louis Jerecki was a security guard for Central State, who still occasionally does work on the vacant and eerie campus.

> What you have to understand is that I hear them all the time. Anybody could. You have to be perceptive, but you can definitely hear them. You hear them on the grounds. There is crying—sometimes screaming, like you used to hear when the patients were still here. While I worked here, we had patients who would scream constantly and who suffered. We even had one patient who hung himself. Sometimes at night you can still hear them scream and moan.

Patient-on-patient violence was common in this area, with the most famous being the story of a patient who was stoned to death by another patient. It is said, as you pass under these trees, that his screams of terror and pain can be heard echoing into the night. In Dan T. Hall's sublime documentary, *Central State Asylum For The Insane*, a former staff member speaking under the condition of anonymity, revealed that the grove of trees holds more than just a few scary stories.

> There's actually two that I knew, patients who had died out there. When I'd go to check the grounds at night when I was a supervisor, I would see shadows move. That just kind of scared me.

Alvin

Perhaps the most famous ghost story to come out of Central State is the story of Alvin, a patient who one day abruptly vanished. He was a minimum security risk and would wander all over the campus. While he posed no risk to the public or himself, a meticulous search was launched, but to no avail. Alvin had simply disappeared and many believed that he had wandered into the streets of Indianapolis. Some years later, a female patient named Agnes began to cut away from her group. She was always found in the same place: seated near the top of the basement steps where all of the violent offenders were kept. When confronted, Agnes told a nurse that she was only talking to her friend, Alvin; that she liked going there to talk with him. "He says he lives in the tunnels," she had said, referring to the intricate system of underground tunnels just six feet away.

Believing that this may have been the same Alvin who had gone missing, another search was launched in an attempt to find the wayward patient. Again, Alvin wasn't found, until one of the pursuing attendants found an open crawl space and looked inside. He immediately found the decomposing body of Alvin, who investigators believe had been lying there for months.

But the discovery of Alvin's body brought up another question: how had he died, and how had he gotten into the crawl space? Had another patient murdered him and stowed his body there? Or had he gotten stuck in the crawlspace and died a slow, painful death?

Alvin was perfectly at home talking to Agnes only, and it was only a stone-cold miracle that his body was found at all. But after the discovery of his body, Agnes never again spoke of him, nor was she ever found near the basement steps again.

Alvin's story has all the ear marks of an urban legend run amok. I haven't been able to prove it *didn't* happen, but, then again, I can't prove that it did, either. Patient records are scarce and not every patient death would have received television or newspaper coverage. But it should be noted that just about every legend has some roots in truth.

The Tunnels

As stated before, the tunnels underneath the hospital ran for a total of five miles, and nearly every cell within the tunnels was full much of the time. Criminally insane, violent sociopaths, and physically aggressive patients were housed here in what was considered the maximum security type of ward. The worst of the worst spent time here. Sexually aggressive rapists, violent offenders, and the thoroughly demented were brought here in an effort to segregate them from the less threatening, more vulnerable patients. Suicides were rampant. The occasional patient-on-patient rapes and murders were committed here as well. But interestingly enough, the tunnels were also a favorite spot for the other patients not confined to the basement cells. Playing Hide and Seek, Tag, and other games children might play were favorite preoccupations.

Here, in the tunnels, dark energy mingles with the innocent and the residual, and the result is a boiling cauldron of paranormal activity that is hard to explain away or debunk as coincidence. Electromagnetic fluctuations, EVPs, and unexplained lights and shadows have been captured in incredible numbers in the tunnels. This is the place where Alvin first made himself known to Agnes, who inadvertently led authorities to his corpse. But Alvin was not the only spirit to roam these dank, dark hallways. The corridors are narrow, the light scant, and sounds echo throughout constantly. Many an employee and investigator alike have reported the tormented screams of Central State's former patients, still angst-ridden by their illness, still chained to their fates.

Moans and the sounds of shuffling feet on the dirt floors of the cells have been heard as well. When deep inside the tunnels, the atmosphere can become heavy and thick, making it difficult to breathe. This can be attributed to closeted claustrophobia, but those affected testify to feelings of being watched, even toyed with, as they make their way through the dark.

The Dorms, the Power Building, and the Cemetery

The outlying dormitories have long been a hotbed of activity. Only natural, considering that these were the places most of the patients called home for twenty hours a day. It is almost a certainty that those who perished here still remain, as the overwhelming and heartrending screams of total madness can still be heard in these chilly and desolate hallways. The footsteps of nurses, a residual phenomenon to be sure, have also been heard.

Inside the old Power House, a building that once supplied power to the entire campus, an old woman's screams have been heard, shadows have been seen darting across hallways, and equipment, especially the coal loader, have started and stopped on their own several times.

A maintenance worker, who had fallen asleep inside the Power House, woke to the feeling of a massive grip of hands upon his throat, choking him. In a panic, he jumped up in the darkness and turned on the lights. He saw nothing. After running from the building and trying to regain his composure, he was shocked to discover that there were red hand marks, deep and angry, around his neck.

The Power House has long been considered the most haunted building on the property, according to investigator reports. This is due to the fact that ghosts require energy to manifest, and the Power House, even though it has been shut down for years, still seems to hold enough residual power to keep the spirits as active as possible.

Back when Central State closed down, redevelopment plans went into effect and the plan was to raze some buildings and redevelop the land for commercial or governmental use. But that was before the old cemeteries were discovered. Lost for decades, these cemeteries hold the remains of Central State's first patients who died while incarcerated. They were subsequently buried in graves marked only with a number in one of two locations: in the northwest corner of the property, and along the western edge of the property near the Pathology Building. The cemetery plots in the Northwest corner are all unmarked, whereas the ones nearest the Pathology Building, while marked, wallow in severe decay, damage, and overgrowth. Still these graves were able to significantly affect the plans the City of Indianapolis had for redeveloping the area.

As of 2010, the cemeteries still stand, the bodies remain, and the soil, thankfully, lies undisturbed. A stone memorial, overgrown with foliage and trees, stands at the entrance of the Northwest cemetery that lists the names of those unfortunate souls buried there. But it is a silent and forgotten memorial that deserves to be seen and appreciated, not hidden away behind fences and brush. For far too long, these unfortunates have been ignored and forgotten when their lives are just as vital and as important as our own.

Psychic Impressions

The immediate impression I received when arriving at Central State Mental Institution's campus was of a blanket – a thick, heavy blanket made up of extreme sadness and pain. It envelops you when you arrive and you feel it immediately. I made two initial visits to the old campus, each one more productive than the last.

The first place to pull on my energy was the Bahr Building, built in 1974. Housing the criminally insane, the Bahr Building drew me to it so hard that I found it difficult to walk away. The doors and windows were locked up tight and what was essentially a nine-foot-tall "moat" surrounded much of the property on the dorm room side. On my first visit to Central State, I felt the pull of a female spirit, but I resisted it and tried to shirk her off as soon as I felt her presence. But the spiritual energy was so strong in that one building that, if I could have found a way in, its doubtful I would ever have been able to leave. It is in that regard that

I quickly began to understand how ghost hunters could become addicted to their favorite haunts, and how dangerous it is to open yourself to—for lack of a better term—parasitical spirits who want you only for your energy.

When I returned a month later with my mother, sister, and nephew, the voices were calmer, quieter. But the draw to the Bahr Building was stronger and I found myself keeping my distance. The intensity was intimidating, but it paled in comparison to the atmosphere and mood of the Carpentry Building (which I will get into later).

My family was impressed with the Bahr Building, but were adamant about checking out the older buildings, ones that were built very early on in the life of this dour place. I immediately led them toward the Administration Building.

We'd found an open door and gladly stepped inside to wander about the ruins, and I was thankful that the atmosphere seemed lighter to me, not as *in-your-face*. What I found especially creepy was the fact that it looked like they had just up and left, leaving paperwork, chairs, magazines, and office supplies strewn everywhere. I was just much more comfortable in that building than I was in the Bahr Building.

Returning to the Carpentry Building, where I had heard the voices on my previous visit, we found a way into the building itself. I was met by the darker energy I had been trying to avoid at the Bahr Building. The air was spotty—cold and warm air mingled freely and hung heavy. My family seemed oblivious to it, so I let them do their thing; my nephew, Eric, did EVP sessions in one room, my mother ruminated about the pain inside a place like this, and my sister drew me toward the darkness.

She found a set of stairs that led down into the basement. What lay in wait down there in the dark is still something that chills my blood. I know that my sister probably noticed how distant I was, and she was right.

A few weeks later, while wandering through my local public library, I came across Lorri Sankowsky and Keri Young's book, *Ghost Hunter's Guide To Indianapolis*. Sankowsky and Young were former co-directors of the Indiana Ghost Trackers, a statewide club of paranormal enthusiasts who I had always admired, yet kept my distance from because I always tended to prefer investigating alone. I'd never laid eyes on the book before and never even thought that Central State might be profiled in it. Lo and behold, Central State was featured prominently in Chapter One.

A chill ran up my spine as I read about their investigation. Mind you, I hadn't seen this book, read about it, nor did I ever meet with the Indiana Ghost Trackers in my life. Keep that in mind, for what they found corroborated my experiences at Central State.

Sankowsky and Young's group had initiated an EVP session in one of the dormitories. Up until that point, they had been thrilled at the number of pictures they'd taken that contained orbs and other light anomalies. But at the conclusion of their EVP session, they played back the recording and were astonished by what they heard. "After several minutes of silence," wrote Sankowsky, "a whispered, drawn out 'no' could be heard, followed by more silence and then what sounded like 'We [or maybe you] shouldn't be here.'"

I was immediately reminded of the voice that had asked me, point blank, "What are you doing here?" ...which brings me back to the Carpentry Building.

Sankowsky and Young also detailed their excursions into my new favorite building, focusing on the group's token psychic intuitive. This psychic felt pure and unadulterated apprehension upon entering the Carpentry Building. "When questioned, she couldn't quite tell us what she was afraid of; she just knew that she did not like this place," wrote Sankowsky. The psychic even ventured down into the basement, but was overwhelmed by a stomach-churning sickness that blanketed her as she stepped into the darkness, a darkness that I had been too scared to step into, and now I know, for very good reason. When she had left the building and stepped outside, the sickness went away.

The validation of knowing that I was right about the Carpentry Building, of trusting my gut feelings and letting them guide me, of knowing that the voice I heard wasn't my imagination.... It was all incredibly enlightening and intoxicating. But I look at Central State differently because of those experiences. They were all very personal experiences that I can't prove to the scientific world, but they eased my mind about the existence of spirits at that place of healing and suffering.

It is my conclusion, and the conclusion of many who have experienced the ghosts there, that Central State Mental Hospital in Indianapolis is one of the most haunted places in the world. It is not a joyride, thrill ride, or circus sideshow. There was a darkness in that place that I wasn't yet comfortable with. It was stronger than I had imagined and it had taken me by surprise, reminding me that this wasn't my ballgame. It was theirs, and it always has been.

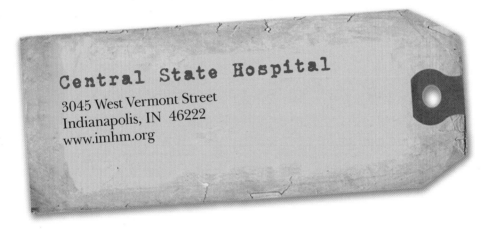

Central State Hospital
3045 West Vermont Street
Indianapolis, IN 46222
www.imhm.org

The Central State campus is open to the public, but owned by the City of Indianapolis. Urban exploration is strongly discouraged, as vagrants and gangs have been known to populate the abandoned buildings from time to time. Private security patrols the grounds at night. I strongly urge anyone interested in investigating Central State to get the cooperation of the police and caretakers on the premises. The unstable buildings aren't the only things at Central State that are hazardous to your health...

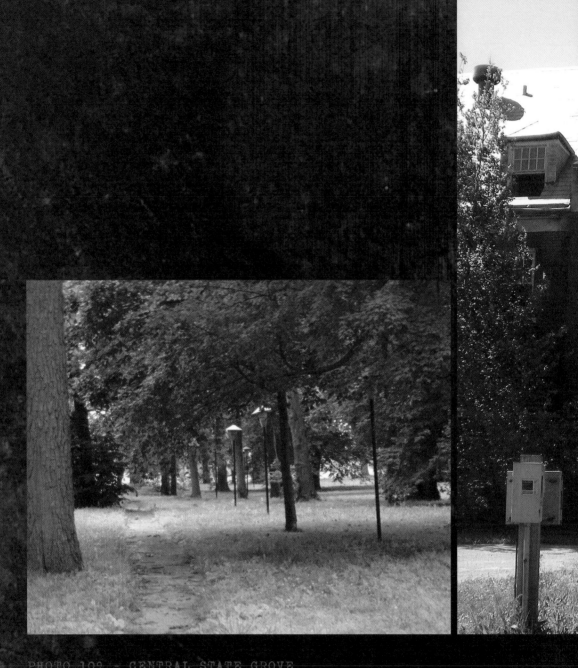

PHOTO 109 - CENTRAL STATE GROVE
On dark nights, Shadow People and the plaintive wailing of anguished souls fill this thick grove of trees near where the original "Seven Steeples" building once stood. *Photo courtesy of the author*.

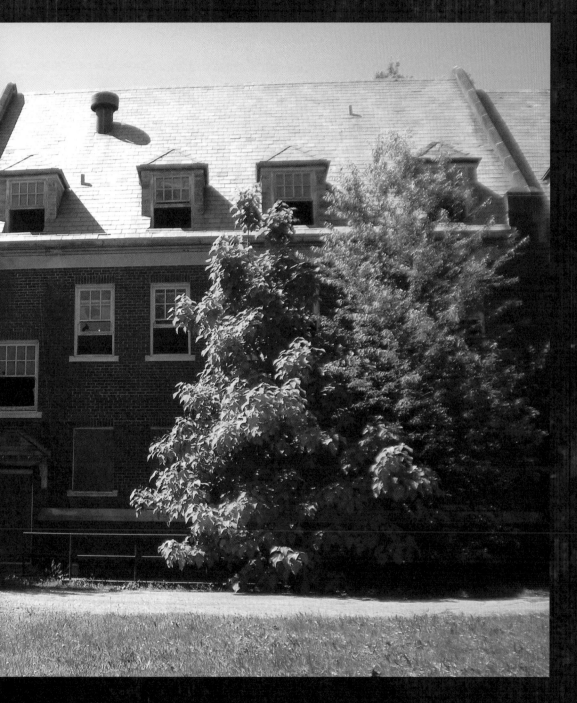

PHOTO 85 - CENTRAL STATE - ADMIN BLDG
The Administration building, one of the only remaining structures of the original Kirkbride-inspired building. It is also said to be one of the more haunted ones. *Photo courtesy of the author.*

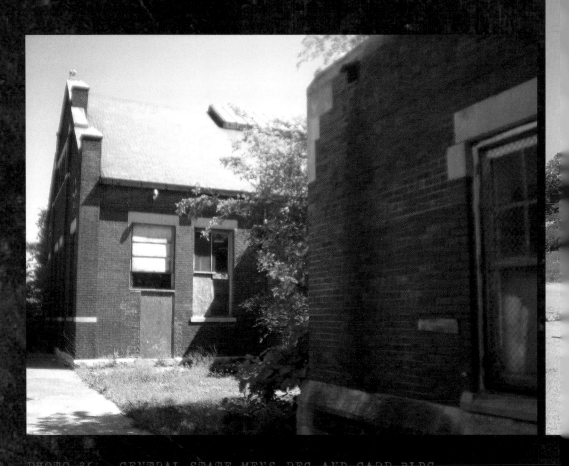

This photo of the Men's Recreation and Carpentry buildings was taken moments before a disembodied voice asked me, "What are you doing here?" *Photo courtesy of the author.*

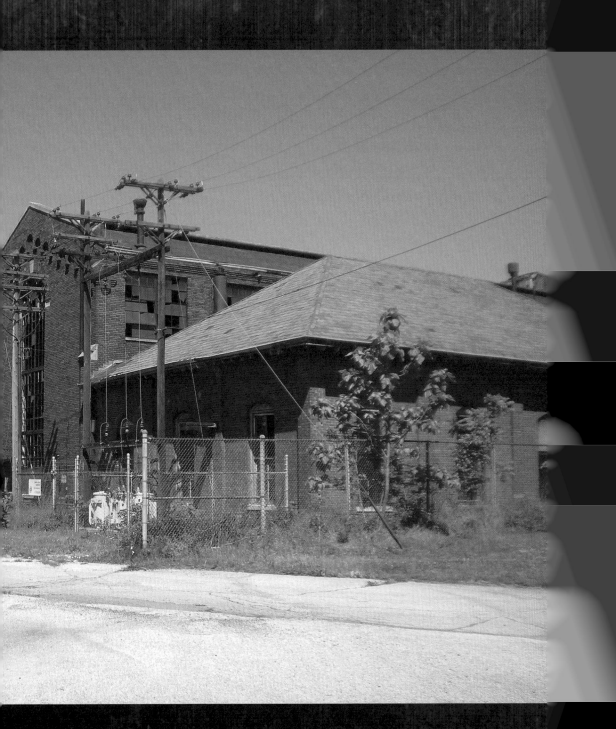

12.

OHIO STATE REFORMATORY
Mansfield, Ohio
1910-1995

"And I did wonder—because it's now three years ago since I left prison—whether there would come a time when I would forget it, or it would be in the past as anything else might be—no, it's there every day of my life."

~Jeffrey Archer

In the small town of Mansfield, Ohio, nestled midway between the bustling metropolis of Akron and Columbus, stands a stone Goliath of thick walls and towering cell blocks. It is here, in this most unassuming of locations, where a tornado of paranormal activity swirls and engulfs the hardy and foolhardy alike. Trapped in places such as The Hole, Cell 13, and a prison graveyard containing the bodies of 215 prisoners not claimed by family, these souls hunger for contact with the living, making themselves known in both benign and malicious ways. Prisons are notorious for retaining negative energy and allowing the souls trapped inside to feast on a steady diet of horror, mayhem, brutality, and melancholy. At the Ohio State Reformatory, there is an endless supply of just that.

But there is a difference between the prison in Mansfield, and the other prisons listed in this book. The spirits there are malicious and evil, hostile and confrontational. A darkness sweeps across the Ohio State Reformatory that has seldom been seen in places other than nightmares and horror movies.

Built between 1886 and 1910 by Levi T. Scofield, a Cleveland architect, and Superintendent F.F. Schnitzer, the hulking Romanesque castle was specifically designed to rehabilitate first-time offenders, and was initially applauded as a positive step toward prison reform. At first, it was supposed to be a boys reformatory for juvenile delinquents, the second step after the Boys Industrial School in Lancaster, and the last step before the harsh reality of the adult Ohio Penitentiary in Columbus.

During the first part of the 20th century, however, the Federal government reinstated the reformatory as a federal corrections center that housed the widest variety of criminals from all over the country. Murderers, rapists, thieves, mobsters, and the like all called Mansfield their home. And even without Death Row, the Ohio State Reformatory still managed to collect over 200 souls, victims of heinous murders and ghastly suicides. Some of those souls belonged to corrections officers, and one is said to be that of a former warden's wife, Helen Glattke.

Between the years 1935 and 1959, Arthur Lewis Glattke was the superintendent in charge of the prison. A well-liked man amongst the guards, as well as the inmates, his ideas of prison reform included piped-in radio music within the cell blocks. But it was Glattke's wife, Helen Bauer Glattke, who has become the star of this tale.

In November of 1950, Helen had been reaching into a jewelry box in the living quarters of the prison when a nearby gun apparently discharged and shot her in the chest. Three days later, she contracted pneumonia during her recuperation and died. Her restless spirit is said to wander the now-empty halls of the warden's quarters.

Initially promising, the Ohio State Reformatory quickly spiraled down into a whirlpool of deplorable conditions, its legacy becoming synonymous with prisoner abuse, torture, and murder. Former inmates still recall appalling conditions that included incredible numbers of rats, vermin, revolting food, and rampant disease. Violence among prisoners, like most prisons, was a way of life as inmates succumbed to shank attacks, beatings, or falls from the towering six-story cell blocks.

In 1948, two deeply disturbed and genuinely evil men were released from OSR on the grounds of good behavior. Robert Daniels and John West, the "Mad Dog Killers," celebrated their release by going on a ruthless killing spree. Their victims included local tavern owner Earl Ambrose, the OSR farm superintendent and his family, a farmer, and a truck driver before they were finally cornered by police. West was shot dead by police, but Daniels was apprehended and eventually died in the electric chair at the Columbus State Penitentiary in 1950.

Ohio State Reformatory had become a haven for brutality, absolute horror, and incredibly thick clouds of dread. It had become the place no one wanted to end up, and it housed brutal, misogynistic, and confrontational men who continually fed their dark energies into this gruesome testament to the depravity of the criminal mind. Eventually, after ninety-four years of operation, in 1990, the Ohio State Reformatory was officially shut down.

The imposing architecture startled and intrigued Hollywood, when, in 1975, *Harry and Walter Go To New York* was filmed there, as was 1988's *Tango & Cash*. But it is probably best known as the dour, grey, bleak façade of Shawshank Prison in Frank Darabont's adaptation of Stephen King's *The Shawshank Redemption* and also the oppressive Soviet prison from *Air Force One*. The state had been looking to demolish the buildings and put the valuable land on the market. But in 1995, shortly after the film opened, ownership of the prison was assumed by The Mansfield Preservation Society.

Considered a blight by most, the prison eventually became renowned and revered by ghost hunters who visited. In the wake of numerous orb photographs and chillingly explicit EVPs, the Ohio State Reformatory began its new life as, in the words of some, the Holy Grail of paranormal hot spots.

The Warden's Quarters

Situated in front of the prison is the cozy outpost of the Warden's Quarters, completely sealed off from the rest of the prison, but close enough for the Warden to respond to crises within the prison. Even this unassuming home has seen its share of death and tragedy, beginning with the death of Warden Glattke's wife. As mentioned earlier, Helen Glattke was suspiciously shot in the chest by a handgun that seemed to discharge as she rummaged through her things. Three years later, Warden Glattke himself became part of the prison's legend by yielding to a massive heart attack in his office. Today, paranormal investigators report hearing voices within the Warden's Quarters. The male and female voices are believed to be the Residual Haunting of Warden Glattke and his wife, their voices raised and heated.

Similarly, the spectral vision of Helen Glattke has been seen in her second-floor sitting room, commonly known as The White Room. The robust smell of roses signal her arrival and she has been known to clearly and politely speak to the living through EVPs. When museum staff threw a party in her honor, she responded to them through EVPs with a polite, sincere "thank you."

In addition to the phantom voices, Warden Glattke's solitary footsteps can be heard strolling through the Administration Wing, courtyards, and living quarters, his discerning eye still inspecting the prison grounds.

The Cell Blocks

It should go without saying that the cell blocks are active with paranormal goings-on. Eerie reports of being touched, usually as visitors walk past the open cell doors, have been described as feeling like a blanket of soft, silky spider webs have floated down into their faces. But with no spider webs to be found, one can only imagine if this is what it feels like when a ghost reaches out for you and actually makes physical contact.

However, touches from the spirits of Mansfield don't always come in the form of soft, velvety strokes. Compared to the cell block areas, the Warden's Quarters is a walk in the park. Here, the spirits are active and hostile, in your face, and definitely not afraid of the living. Aggression is rampant here, especially when the victim of such attacks are female or elderly. Female museum workers, tour guides, and elderly patrons have reported their hair getting pulled, punches, and slaps to the body and head, and the disturbing sensation of disembodied breathing on the backs of their necks.

Here in the cell blocks, EVPs come in the form of blatant vulgarity, defiance, and challenges, a trait not unlike their living counterparts from long ago. The sounds of screams, footsteps, slamming cell doors, and aggressive threats of violence have all been captured by various ghost hunters and paranormal researchers.

It is also in these cell blocks that the majority of shadow figures, mists, and orbs are photographed. "There were five of us here (in East Block,)" says Susan Nicole, Operations Manager for OSR. "And we heard a bang clear down where the cells bow out a little bit. And we saw a figure, a whitish figure, lean out, and then back up really quickly."

Also equally distressing are the tales of people being violently pushed from behind, as in the case of one anonymous woman who was touring the prison's annual Halloween haunted house. She and a group of high school friends had begun to head down a set of rickety stairs and as she brought up the rear behind the students, she was violently pushed from behind, causing her to fall to one knee. But when she turned to look, she found no one there.

Shadow People also figure into the legend of Ohio State Reformatory, for it is on the East Cell Block's third tier that shuffling figures can be seen in the darkness, languidly moving from cell door to cell door, disappearing and reappearing as white and dark mists, their forms becoming one with the darkness before your very eyes. They will walk back and forth between the railings and the cells, almost as if pacing, as if watching or waiting for someone—*anyone*—to return.

From one floor above, on the fourth tier of East Block, comes a tale of a prisoner who, after all hope had abandoned him, brought a bed sheet out of his cell during line-up for lunch call. As each prisoner joined the line, this hopeless man tied one of the ends of the sheet around his neck and the other end around the railing. With nary a breath upon his lips, he jumped over the fourth-floor railing, hanging himself for the entire cell block to see.

Now, during some of the more recent ghost hunts, investigators claim to have seen the white apparition of a man hanging from the fourth-floor railing, his misty, lifeless body swaying slowly back and forth.

Lockhart

In Cell 13, on the fourth floor of East Cell Block, a weary, hopeless spirit re-lives his final hours, over and over and over again. His pain has become a badge that the OSR wears whether it wishes to or not. His full name is lost to legend now, but possibly the most famous—or infamous—prisoner in the OSR is a man now known only as Lockhart.

Assigned to Cell 13, Lockhart was a solitary man whose family had all but disowned him for the crimes he had committed.

No one knows for certain what finally drove Lockhart to suicide, but the lingering air of depression and hopelessness that ran through the walls and halls of the OSR probably had as much to do with it as Lockhart's own mental issues. Smuggling a can of paint thinner from one of the prison's machine shops, Lockhart made his way back to his cell where a lone stick match lay waiting. Who knows what went through his mind as he doused himself with the paint thinner and struck the match? Immediately, the entire cell block was awash in the sound of Lockhart's screams and the smell of his burning flesh.

When he was finally pulled from his cell, Lockhart was still smoldering and great pieces of cooked flesh were falling from his bones, trailing behind him as he was dragged from the cell block and to the infirmary.

Today, people still see a shadowy figure inside Lockhart's old Cell 13. They sometimes hear his screams; other times they feel a dark, heavy presence of sadness or anger. Increasingly rarer are the smells of fire and burning flesh that once wafted through the cell block during Lockhart's self-inflicted immolation.

One has to wonder: what finally drove Lockhart to such gruesome extremes? Medium Lynne Olson has pointed a finger at the presence of a darker, more diabolical entity that held sway over Lockhart, even controlled him by manipulating his moods, attitude, and thoughts. But was Lockhart's suicide the end result of a demon's plan? Or was it the final, desperate act of a man wanting to sever ties with his demonic tormentor?

The Hole

Like every other prison in the world, the OSR has its own set of cell blocks away from the general population. Located in the darker recesses of the lower prison, Solitary Confinement gave new definition to the term. Only the most outrageous, angry, and defiant men were sent to The Hole. Conceivably, the most horrifying expectation for all prisoners was "The Hole," or Solitary Confinement. These cells were outfitted with nothing but a toilet, a bunk, and infinite darkness.

Prisoners would spend days, even months in these cells for any variety of infraction, ranging from insubordination to murder.

There were twenty solitary confinement cells on the lower levels of OSR, and following a riot in the 1930s, 120 prisoners were confined to "The Hole" for 30 days, making the count a staggeringly deplorable 10 people per cell. Surprisingly, when they were all finally released from The Hole, only one inmate had been killed, his body hidden under bedding by the others.

In another instance of brutality, a convict bludgeoned a guard to death with an iron bar during an escape attempt that originated in The Hole. His authoritative footsteps are still heard, not just in The Hole, but around the cell blocks as well. Today, it should come as no surprise that The Hole is the most active part of the OSR, with spirits as mean and aggressive in the afterlife as they were in their former lives. Elderly people and women seem to be the biggest targets, enduring punches, slaps, hair pulling, and taunting voices that range from threatening to vulgar.

Women especially have endured quite a few taunts and touches, ranging from the harmless yet thoroughly creepy stroking of their hair to having their heads shoved downward by invisible hands. Some women have had their buttocks grabbed, and others have been whispered to suggestively. In a prison that once housed only men and employed no women, the idea of a sweet-smelling female is still a powerful trigger object for these lonely spirits, which makes women the best bait possible when conducting a ghost hunt.

Interestingly enough, when I toured the prison in May 2012, I performed an impromptu EVP session in Solitary. This was the only place where I could actually do an EVP session; the tours of the other places were so cram-packed with loud, talkative people that doing an EVP session with a group of forty and a tour guide would have been next to impossible. But being alone in Solitary Confinement with only a bulldozer working outside and no other *living* souls on the block, I was able to do a quick little session that yielded an interesting result.

I was walking through Solitary, asking the spirits, "Is there anyone in Solitary here with me? Or am I alone?" No answer. But when I played the voice file back on my computer, I heard a very distinctive female voice say, "Promise?" A short time later in the session, I asked, "What is your name?" Moments passed before a very faint, breathy voice, the same voice I'd heard before on the digital voice recorder, responded, "Helllllen."

This was proof positive to me that I had been in contact with the ghost of Helen Glattke, the only known female spirit said to haunt the OSR. She had even identified herself by name, which made it hard for anyone to dispute. The only issue was that it was spoken so softly that many people who listened to it didn't hear it. This is a common hindrance to the lay person, as it can take years to train your hearing to pick up even the softest whisper hidden in the white noise of an audio file.

During the Halloween season, the OSR traditionally serves as a "Spook House," complete with costumed actors and special effects. It has been said that, as patrons wander through the haunted attraction, they report being extremely frightened by a number of men who other workers have never met, mostly in Solitary Confinement. These men are never seen again and are never accounted for by the other staged haunt workers.

During the other parts of the year, the OSR hosts daylight and overnight ghost hunts for a nominal fee, with all proceeds going to the funds needed to fully restore the OSR.

Psychic Impressions

According to medium Tina Michelle, an intense energy swells inside the Ohio State Reformatory. While most of the Solitary Confinement cells resonate with darkness, surprisingly, the remaining spirits just wanted to be heard. Many lost souls cried out to her for help in crossing over, which she claims she did with the help of her guides.

The most overwhelming impression she received is fairly tragic and melancholy: the spirits are both angry and sad about either being left behind or voluntarily remaining on Earth because they fear God's judgment. Amongst the majority of the spirits, there is an urgent need to be remembered and for their stories to be told.

Medium Lynne Olson addressed the somewhat misogynistic attitudes the spirits have toward women who work at the prison, particularly those spirits that reside in Solitary. Unlike the rest of the prison where the spirits tend to be former prisoners, Olson says that Solitary holds an eclectic mix of spirits that are both inmates and guards. In death as in life, they stand on opposite sides of the bars like rival gangs on the same turf. But there is a shared philosophy amongst them. They both seem to enjoy their brutality, their freedom to do whatever they want to whomever they want, and the warm and fuzzy feeling of being able to get away with it. It is this group of renegade, dangerous spirits that taunt and terrorize the female staff at the Ohio State Reformatory and there are only a few who wish to protect them. When you go to visit the OSR, hopefully, you'll catch the eye of one of the good ones.

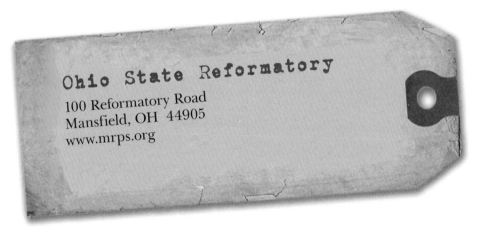

Ohio State Reformatory
100 Reformatory Road
Mansfield, OH 44905
www.mrps.org

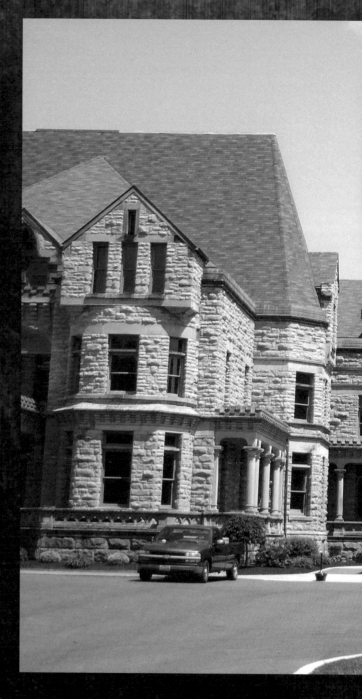

The Ohio State Reformatory in Mansfield, Ohio. *Photo courtesy of the author.*

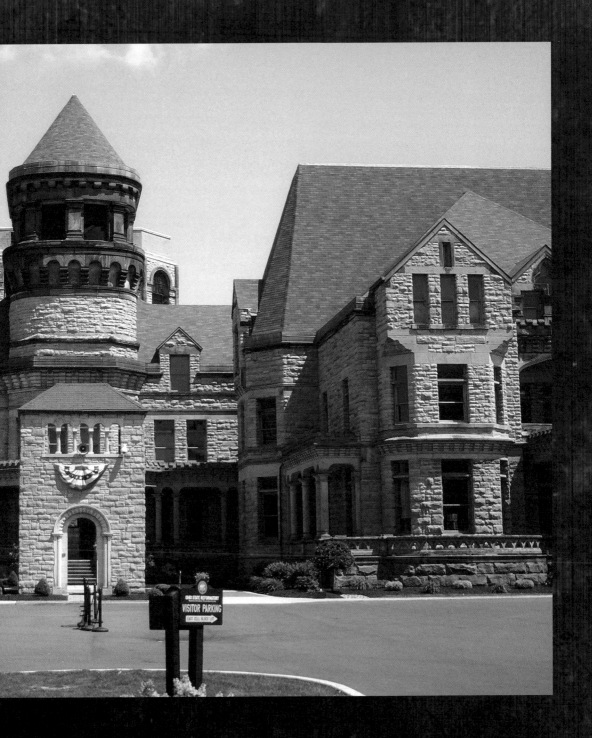

OHIO STATE REFORMATORY
VISITOR PARKING
EAST CELL BLOCK LOT

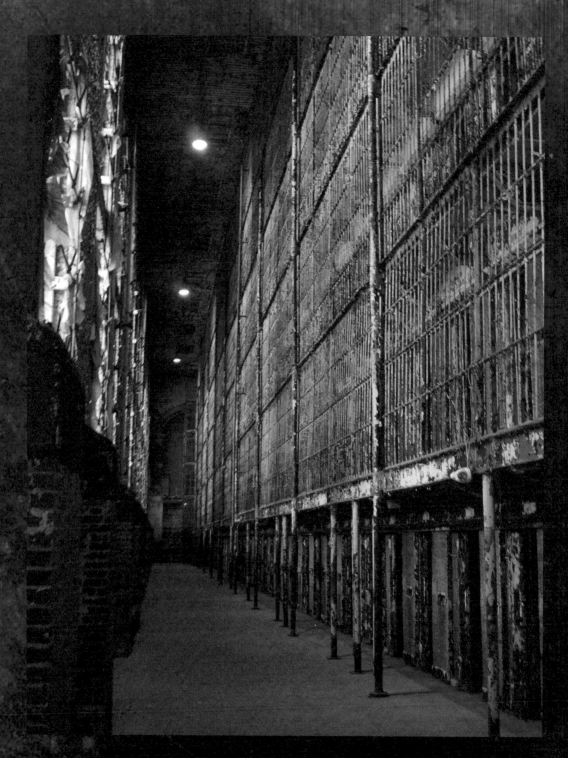

PHOTO 93 - OHIO STATE REFORMATORY 016
Standing six tiers high, the Ohio State Reformatory boasts the largest free-standing steel prison in the world. *Photo courtesy of the author.*

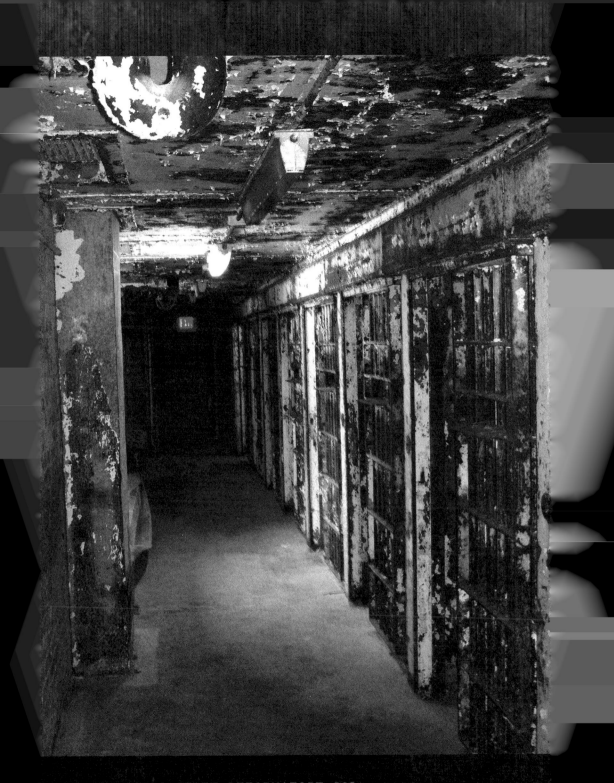

PHOTO 94 - OHIO STATE REFORMATORY 021
The dank and sinister Solitary Confinement, where I captured an EVP of who I believe was
Helen Glattke, a former warden's wife who is said to haunt the prison. *Photo courtesy of the*

13.

ALCATRAZ FEDERAL PENITENTIARY
San Francisco, California
1934-1964

"Hope is the worst of evils, for it prolongs the torment of man."

~Friedrich Nietzsche

Alcatraz is, without a doubt, the most famous prison in the world. Its stone cells held the most famous gangsters and criminals the world has ever seen. Machine Gun Kelly, Robert Stroud, and Al Capone all spent time here. It is one of the most recognizable landmarks in the United States. Each year, millions of tourists flock to it and marvel at the mystique of Alcatraz.

The irony isn't lost on the spirits. When they were alive, they wanted nothing more than to be able to leave "The Rock." But now people are taking boats and paying to get inside. Capone and his buddies must be shaking their heads, either in disgust or disbelief.

Whatever the case, Alcatraz Federal Penitentiary has earned, deserves, and retains its title of the most effective and disciplined prison in the world. Nicknamed "The Rock" because of the rocky island foundation upon which the prison was built, it offered little to no hope for escape, and mercy was no longer in the vernacular of convict and guard alike.

Movies and television shows have glamorized it, but the reality of Alcatraz is drab, miserable, solid, and unforgiving.

Alcatraz began its life as a useless island in the San Francisco Bay; its foundations, made of granite, made it impossible to sustain any kind of life. The first to find use for the tiny island was the American military who, in 1847, realized how pertinent it was to maintaining a good watch over one of the busiest harbors on the West Coast. America's enemies could be spotted and stopped well before gaining any real foothold on American soil. By 1853, the first military installation on Alcatraz was completed. The fortress featured several long-range cannons, as well as four enormous 36,000-pound Rodman guns, capable of sinking ships up to three miles away. Incidentally, soldiers on Alcatraz fired one of the cannons only once and missed the target completely. However, its reputation as an icon of American military power was undeniable.

As the years went on, the armaments on Alcatraz began to show their age as new, more modern weapons overtook the military conscience. Added to that was the waning need for a military installation, as other, more secure fortresses were dreamed and realized. It was at that point that the military realized Alcatraz's worth as a stockade. Being frigid in the winter and shark infested in the summer, the choppy waters provided an incredible deterrent to escape attempts and work began on converting Alcatraz from a military fortress to a military prison. They began receiving prisoners of the Civil War in 1861. Then, with the advent of the Spanish-American War, their population rose from a mere 26 prisoners to an astounding 450. Word got around quickly that "The Rock" was as close to Hell as one could get without getting burned.

Prisoners who violated the rules were subject to hard-labor work details wearing the now-iconic ball and chain, and enduring days or months at time being locked down in solitary confinement, usually with a strict bread and water diet. Interestingly enough, the prison cells were used only for sleeping. Unless the prisoner was on lock-down, all convicts were prohibited from visiting their cells during the day and were allowed to roam anywhere on the prison grounds, excepting of course the guards quarters on the upper levels. No matter what crime the convict had been convicted of, he was still a soldier in the United States military and the lax security was a luxury afforded to them. A few tried to take advantage of the lenient security by making a break for it, trying to swim across the San Francisco Bay. But either the freezing waters made them turn back, or tired them out so much that they drowned. Either way, the point was well taken by the convicts, who quickly saw escape as a no-win situation.

Rising operational costs forced the Department of War to abandon Alcatraz, bequeathing it to the Department of Justice, who reopened it in 1934 as a maximum security penitentiary. All of the cell blocks were reinforced. The infirmary and solitary cells were renovated. Nicknamed Uncle Sam's Devil's Island, Alcatraz quickly became known as the final stop for many of America's most dangerous criminals. Gone was the lax security and nearly-boundless freedoms afforded to the military's prisoners. In its place was a rigid series of rules, regulations, and routines that broke each convict down to his most primal state and rebuilt him in the image of discipline and compliance.

Each prisoner would receive his own cell. Contact with the outside world was severed almost completely. Mail was opened, read, and censored before convicts would receive it. Inmates weren't allowed to explore the cell houses; instead, they were marched from one location to another in a cohesive formation reminiscent of the military that used to populate the island. Privileges could be earned, but taken away just as quickly should the rules be violated in any way. Not even Al Capone, arguably the most famous and influential gangster of all time, received any special privileges. Jailed for tax evasion and transferred to Alcatraz, it was made very clear that the privileges he had been used to in other prisons would not be available to him at Alcatraz. That never stopped him from trying to gain special attention, but eventually he conceded defeat, saying, "It looks like Alcatraz has got me licked."

Another famous prisoner was also Alcatraz's unofficial mascot. Robert Stroud, the so-called "Birdman Of Alcatraz" was one of the few inmates who spent his entire incarceration in the Alcatraz Segregation Unit. This was due to the fact that Stroud had been an extraordinarily volatile and hostile prisoner toward guards and fellow convicts alike as he served time at Leavenworth Prison in Kansas. Rather than risk harm or give such a violent man an opportunity to cause ripples in the rigid routine, he was never once introduced into the general population of Alcatraz. While at Leavenworth, Stroud developed a keen interest in birds, keeping up a roost and tending to his feathered friends whenever he could. But when he was sent to Alcatraz, he was immediately prohibited from keeping any birds while incarcerated. Stroud spent six years in isolation in D Block, and eleven in the prison hospital. In 1959, *The Birdman of Alcatraz*, starring Burt Lancaster as Stroud, was released and Stroud's celebrity became mythic. His fan mail increased significantly, enough to infuriate and frustrate the censors who had to peruse each letter before sending it on to Stroud. The film and the Stroud character were so popular that thousands lobbied for Stroud's release.

That, of course, did not happen. Alcatraz and Leavenworth officials knew what Robert Stroud was: a thrice convicted murderer with a volatile personality and a taste for young children. He reveled in his celebrity status and found a sick amusement to it all. As one inmate later commented, "They want to free Burt Lancaster, not Robert Stroud." He was a brutal, incredibly intelligent psychopath who attacked whenever he had the opportunity and may have been responsible for inciting a riot that lasted for three solid days.

Later that year, Stroud was transferred out of Alcatraz to the Medical Center for Federal Prisoners in Springfield, Missouri. He died of natural causes just four years later on November 21, 1963. It wasn't too much later, in 1964, that Alcatraz closed its doors for good, the reasons being a substantial lack of funding to remain operational.

As is what happens when an era ends, those who either lived it or survived it began to exchange stories and tales about "The Rock." Everyone wanted to hear Capone stories, but once word got out that Alcatraz just might be haunted, the public began to clamber for more. And "The Rock" had many tales to tell.

Solitary Cell 14

If you were to ask a prison guide about the most strange and haunting tale to come out of Alcatraz, most likely you would hear the story of Cell 14, a solitary confinement cell in D Block. Even to this day, Cell 14 stays colder than the rest of the prison, almost requiring a jacket if you were to spend any quality time in there. It's even colder than the other three solitary cells, and there is a strange, almost ghostly intensity that radiates out from it.

In the mid-1940s, an inmate had been banished to The Hole for violating one of the rules. Standard procedure, as it were. Within seconds of being locked inside Cell 14, the inmate began to scream in terror. According to the inmate, a creature with glowing red eyes had been locked in with him. His story was ignored and the door was shut once more.

The inmate continued to scream throughout the night until a deathly silence finally began to saturate The Hole. The next day, guards inspected the cell and discovered that the inmate was dead, a terrified expression frozen onto his face. Around his neck were unmistakable red handprints. An autopsy had concluded that the inmate had not only died of strangulation, but was strangled so badly that it would have been impossible to do it upon himself. It is possible that one of the guards had choked him to quiet him down. Still others believe it may have been the spirit of a former inmate out to avenge himself on the one who killed him.

As the guards and inmates were trying to unravel the mystery for themselves, the day following the inmates strangulation, several guards were performing their routine head count and noticed there were too many men in the lineup. At the end of the line, they saw the face of the inmate who had been strangled to death in Cell 14. Stunned, the guards and inmates looked on as the figure dissipated from view.

To this day, visitors and investigators alike have felt a dark, heavy presence in Cell 14 of D Block. One visitor recalled being accosted in the darkness of Cell 14 by something that grabbed his shoulder and whispered in his ear,

"You're mine." The boy, 14 at the time, would carry this trauma with him for most of his life. The Alcatraz episode of The Travel Channel's *The Dead Files* went on to profile this man, with acclaimed psychic medium Amy Allan confirming the man's story that a dark entity still roamed D Block, one that was full of pain and astoundingly angry.

So who is the spirit that roams D Block? It could be that of the psychotic Robert Stroud, who spent the better part of his time on Alcatraz in The Hole. But what is certain is that a dark presence has definitely lodged itself in that cell and whatever lives there doesn't live alone.

The Ghost of Robert Stroud

Robert Stroud enjoyed his celebrity status in life and now revels in it in death. Still contained inside Alcatraz, he watches as visitors and tourists explore his old stomping grounds. Those who have seen Robert Stroud's ghost report the same thing: an older man dressed in his prison clothes. His presence is almost always accompanied by a gust of cold air and, occasionally, the smell of bath soaps that he favored during his daily bath.

In life, Stroud was a flippant, unpredictable madman, and most psychics who have visited in the past say that Stroud walks about Alcatraz like a king, taunting visitors and becoming enraged when disrespected in even the slightest ways. Those who see his residual imprint see the madness firsthand. Amy Allan even referred to him as "Monkey Man" because of the wild and bizarre nature of his in-cell ranting.

Some things never change.

The Sounds of Sadness

The most common, and heartbreaking, paranormal experiences have been heard and not seen. From different areas of the prison, the sounds of sobbing and weeping echo. No one has been able to explain or debunk these sounds of sadness. Admittedly, crying and sobbing would be commonplace on occasion from some of the newer convicts, but no source of the crying could ever be found. Such a common occurrence this was that even Warden Johnston, an avowed skeptic, commented on it to his subordinates, saying that he heard sobbing coming from within the stone walls. This sound was joined by an unearthly cold that whipped around him furiously.

Warden Johnston thought that someone was lodged in the walls following a possible escape attempt. But when a search and a head count was conducted, all convicts were present and accounted for. It is possible that he believes now.

There were often conversations amongst guards and convicts as well about the sound of crying and moaning, unexplained smells, deathly cold spots, and even full-bodied apparitions of not only prisoners, but soldiers as well, the first convicts of the island. Unexplained gunshots, cannon bursts, and the low voices of men deep in conversation: These sounds resonate throughout Alcatraz, from the bowels of the caverns below to the watch towers on the shore.

Capone and His Banjo?

It sounds like a joke, but it is true. Al Capone, the most famous Sicilian gangster who ever lived, the most brutal, ruthless mobster of recent memory, relaxed by playing his banjo. Of course, one wouldn't dare laugh, giggle, or even grin to Capone's face, for Al took the playing of the banjo very seriously. It brought him peace and harmony in a world where death was as easy to catch as the common cold.

During his last days at Alcatraz, Capone never went outside to partake in recreation time. Years of dodging bullets and knives had made him paranoid, and rightfully so. His age and health was waning and he knew that if a young con shanked the notorious Al Capone, that con's reputation would be set for life. As a result, Al Capone often hid out in the shower room, playing his banjo, having received special permission from the warden. The twinkling of the banjo strings would echo throughout the cell block and some say it still does to this day.

After Capone's death from syphilis in 1947, tour guides and park rangers all began to report hearing the sounds of Al Capone's banjo, the music radiating from the shower room he favored. Although Capone died in his home in Florida, could his ghost be returning to Alcatraz to partake in a little banjo pickin'? Or was his passion for playing so great that it created an imprint on Alcatraz, one that plays on a loop over and over again?

Psychic Impressions

World renowned psychic medium Peter James, perhaps one of the most respected mediums working in the field of the paranormal, once toured Alcatraz Island and was nearly overwhelmed by the hundreds of voices speaking aloud to him all at once. He is convinced that there is an energy on "The Rock" unlike anything he had ever experienced before. Peter James is convinced that there are at least 100 ghosts here still walking the cell block hallways, looking for a way out of their plight. During his walkthrough of Alcatraz, he was particularly drawn to the energies in Cell 403.

Psychic medium Annette Martin also felt the powerful energies in Cell 403 as images of blood, violence, beatings, and feelings of being trapped or caged began to flood her mind. Out of all the places in Alcatraz, it was this place that stuck in her memory the most.

In May of 1946, a convict serving a life term named Bernard Paul Coy and an accomplice named Joseph Cretzer managed to enact an elaborate plan to escape Alcatraz. During a period of time when most of the inmates were busy in the industrial complex of the prison, Coy and Cretzer put their plan into action. Amazingly, they were able to infiltrate one of the guard stations and overwhelm nine guards, placing them into Cell 403 and 404. The escape attempt failed, but not before the guards who were taken hostage had been beaten and locked into the cells.

Obviously, the residual pain of that day still echoes through Alcatraz. Although order and discipline was strictly enforced, the simple fact of the matter was that you could take the animal off the streets, but it doesn't stop being an animal. Assaults, murders, and suicides dotted Alcatraz's history, and the results of that still clamor for attention to this day. The list of paranormal experiences at Alcatraz could fill numerous pages in numerous books. It is a dream location for paranormal investigators and mediums. But for the spirits of Alcatraz, escaping from "The Rock" is easier said than done, even in death.

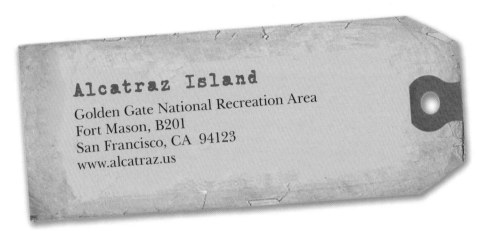

Alcatraz Island
Golden Gate National Recreation Area
Fort Mason, B201
San Francisco, CA 94123
www.alcatraz.us

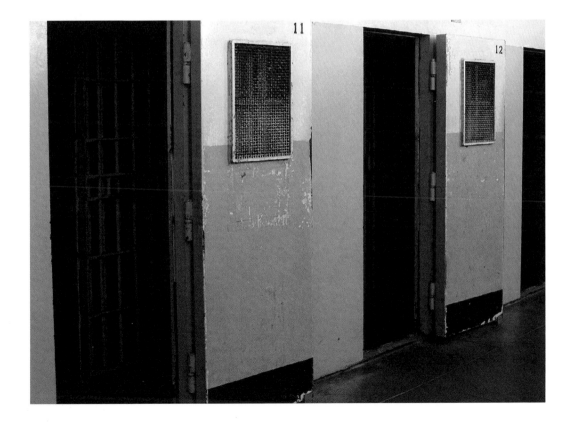

PHOTO 20-ALCATRAZ SOLITARY
Cell block D, the Solitary Confinement unit of Alcatraz. Just a few doors down from here begins one of the most terrifying ghost stories "The Rock" has ever known. *Photo courtesy of Anna Katherine.*

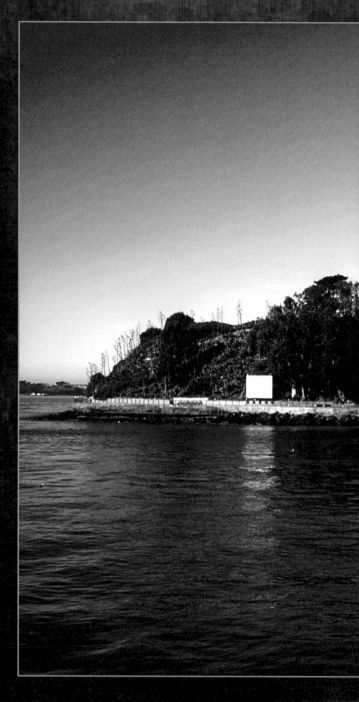

PHOTO 18-ALCATRAZ EXTERIOR
Alcatraz Federal Penitentiary. *Photo courtesy of Anna Katherine.*

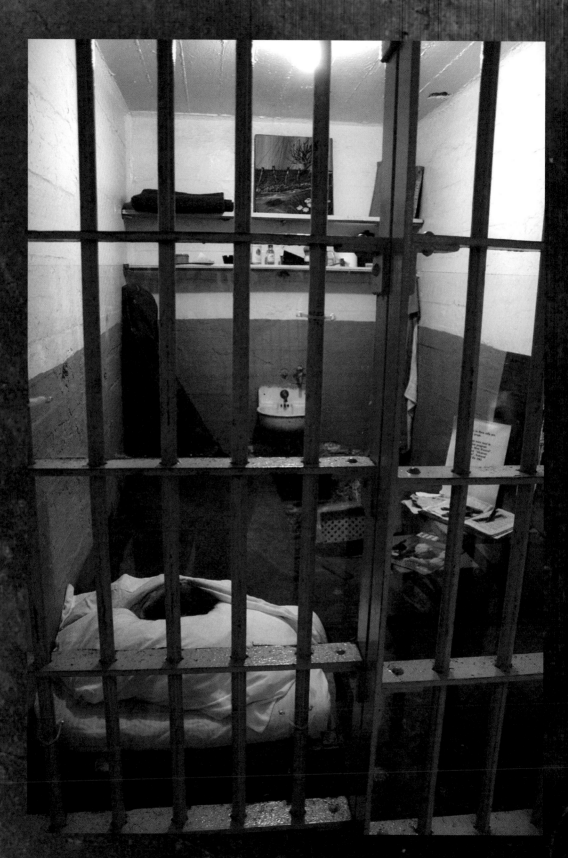

PHOTO 21 ALCATRAZ MODEL CELL
The typical cell in Alcatraz and one very similar to cell #403 and #404. *Photo courtesy of Anna Katherine.*

14.

YORKTOWN MEMORIAL HOSPITAL
Yorktown, Texas
1951-1988

"I don't believe that ghosts are 'spirits of the dead' because I don't believe in death. In the multiverse, once you're possible, you exist. And once you exist, you exist forever one way or another. Besides, death is the absence of life, and the ghosts I've met are very much alive. What we call ghosts are lifeforms just as you and I are."

~Paul F. Eno
Footsteps in the Attic

The idea of the ghosts of former nuns seems a tad ironic, if not genuinely hypocritical of the religious dogma by which all who are faithful to the Christian religion embrace. If those who devoted their lives to God could not, or cannot, receive entry into Heaven, who can? Yet, that is who people in Yorktown, Texas believe haunt this former hospital: the nuns who financed it and had it built.

Yorktown, Texas is really a place of no special significance. Its most famous native was Harlon Block, a soldier in World War II who had the distinction of being one of the men who raised the American flag over Iwo Jima, captured in an iconic photograph that defined the principles of America's role in the War for many people. Its population boasts just over 2,000 people living in a town only 1.7 miles in area.

Opened in 1951, Yorktown Memorial Hospital was financed and built by the nuns of the Roman Catholic order of the Felician Sisters. The nuns had bought the land, built the structures, and staffed it almost entirely themselves with the help of a small crew of doctors, surgeons, and nurses. It was to be a true place of healing under God's wings with the strict Roman Catholic structure lying underneath of it all.

Almost immediately, the hospital began to experience a horrific amount of deaths within the Neo-Natal unit—deaths of children being born without the benefit of Natal Intensive Care Unit equipment. Fragile births at Yorktown, invariably, meant death came quickly for the youngest and most innocent of souls. It has been speculated, yet never proven, that, despite the strong Roman Catholic discipline, abortions were performed semi-regularly and the illegitimate children of rapes and incest cases received little to no medical attention. In short, it was said that the nuns basically let these feeble abominations die. After a time, however, a large cash donation was made to purchase NICU equipment and the rate of child death dropped.

On the second floor of the hospital lay the mental health unit, where victims of paranoid schizophrenia, bi-polar disorder, and even alcoholism and drug abuse were treated. When a slight epidemic of tuberculosis erupted in Yorktown, patients were housed amongst the insane, with the first floor of the hospital reserved for child birth, emergency rooms, and surgical suites. During its thirty-year run, little to no scandals or unsolved mysteries occurred. The hospital existed quietly. But when its doors closed in 1980, stories of ghosts and unexplained sounds began to circulate, even as it reopened in 1981 as a substance abuse clinic. Closed for good in 1988, the stories began to accumulate and its reputation as one of the most haunted hospitals in America began to grow.

The Yorktown Love Triangle

The most famous incident of murder in Yorktown's history supposedly happened in the hospital itself, tucked deep down inside the basement areas. It has been said that a woman employed at the hospital during its time as a substance abuse clinic began an affair with two men, patients receiving treatment for their addictions. While she was carrying on with one man in the basement area, the other caught them both and stabbed each one to death. The bloodstains from this brutal attack are still visible to this day under the intensity of a black light.

Down in the basement, the murder seems to replay over and over again, a classic Residual Haunting that, oddly, becomes an Intelligent Haunting the longer one stays down there. Investigators have heard their own names being called out in the darkness, EVPs of a woman groaning in pain have been captured, and the quick, darting shadows of doomed lovers all come together and relive their shocking deaths night after night.

One thing that always seems to come at paranormal investigators at this location is a barrage of energy that many believe are the spirits of the murdered woman and her lover, energy that seems to want the outside world to know who really killed them. But the answer to that question may be lost to the ages, and a tragic new tale of doomed love has sprung up in its place.

But did the murder even happen at all? No evidence, records, or testimonies exist that would seem to bear witness to the validity of the story of the three doomed lovers. It could have been covered up in an attempt to keep the reputation of Yorktown Memorial from being sullied by the heinous act of double homicide. Yet, compelling evidence has been collected down in the basement that would seem to point to the spirits of a woman and a man. EVPs collected by various investigators have all captured the voice of a woman who warns them that "the killer is coming" and to "hide." K-II meters and EMF detectors light up like Christmas trees in the basement area. The devastating feeling of being watched almost overpowers some investigators. Something roams the basement hallways, and if it is not the spirits of the murdered woman and her lover, then what haunts the basement?

The Nun's Chapel

One wing of the hospital is devoted entirely to the Chapel area, also used as the Nuns' Lounge area. While it was in operation, men were strictly forbidden from entering this place, and those with tattoos were treated in quite a hostile way. According to the nuns who haunt this place, that rule is still in effect. Men who venture into the chapel wing have reported being choked and beaten by unseen forces until they leave the area, and those sporting tattoos of any kind have received similar treatment. Light-headedness, dizziness, and an overwhelming feeling of being watched are some of the more prevalent effects this area of the hospital has on men and tattooed investigators. Despite the absence of electricity in the hospital, K-II meters and EMF detectors light up and prove the existence of energy fields not conducted by wires.

Sightings of dark shadows are plentiful in this section of the hospital, lending credence to the stories that, even in death, the nuns are running their hospital their own way and in accordance with God's law. Maybe the disciplined Mother Superior or another Matron of high distinction has pledged services to maintaining the chapel's integrity. Perhaps that is the reason they stay. It is their duty, their responsibility, to maintain Yorktown Memorial as a place of healing, both in physical and spiritual means. They stay not because they are lost, but because they are the ones who have seen the light and remain to help others find their way.

Yorktown Memorial Hospital is privately owned, and, as of this writing, has been banned by the Yorktown City Council from hosting any kind of public paranormal investigations, sleep overs, or parties. For more information, visit www.yorktownhospital.com.

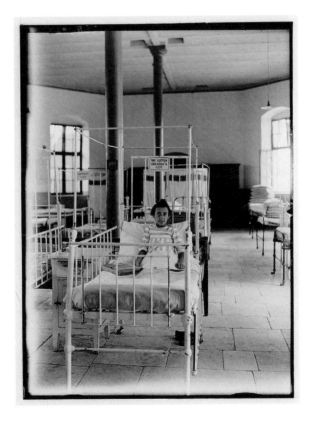

PHOTO 84 GIRL IN HOSPITAL BED

15.

THE TRANS-ALLEGHENY LUNATIC ASYLUM

Weston, West Virginia

1881-1994

"A lot of these people's families have disowned them because of the mental illness. The centers are their families."

~Lee Woodland

The story of a little girl named Lily really grabs your attention here at the Trans-Allegheny Lunatic Asylum, formerly the Weston State Hospital. She now is the spirit of a little girl who died here, abandoned by her parents and forced to live amongst the numerous other orphans who had also been abandoned by their parents. Her story is not unique; it is but one tragedy in a long line of suffering and loss that is all too common in this haunted place, where loneliness reigned and misery was a way of life.

Built between 1858 and 1881, with construction halting only once during the American Civil War, the Weston State Hospital became the largest hand-cut stone building in America, and second in the world next to the Kremlin in Russia. Its sprawling, staggered wings and connecting structures were built specifically to make the most of the available fresh air and sunlight for its patients. Built at first by prison laborers, they were eventually replaced by German and Irish masons, brought to the new world to specifically build this expansive monument to anguish and rehabilitation.

Created to house only 250 patients, the Weston State Hospital reached its apex in the 1950s with over 2,400 patients. This was due mostly to the fact that the values attached to mental rehabilitation were incredibly flexible. Criminally insane men and women were the first to be admitted, but over time, orphans, homosexuals, alcoholics, epileptics, drug addicts, the mentally retarded, derelicts, and any other person that a family might deem undesirable were placed here. No questions asked, no judgment passed.

Over time, a 200-foot clock tower was erected, as well as separate buildings for women and African-Americans. In the end, the hospital became fairly self-sufficient, with a farm, waterworks, dairy, and cemetery, all tended to by patients under the watchful eyes of doctors and nursing staff.

But not all at the Weston State Hospital was rosy and peaceful. One needs to remember that, even with the pleasant diversions listed above, there were barbaric treatments used to control the more violent patients. The most notorious means of control was the ice pick frontal lobotomy. Over the course of the Weston State Hospital's history, over 3,500 lobotomies were performed using a simple ice pick. Instead of common anesthesia, patients were administered electroshock therapy until they were rendered nearly unconscious. With the patient dazed, confused, and docile, an ice pick was inserted between the eyeball and eyelid, punching a hole through the ocular cavity and into the brain itself. Once inside the frontal lobe of the brain, the surgeon would make a sweeping motion with the ice pick, successfully disconnecting the frontal lobe of the brain. Because Weston State Hospital was severely overcrowded and the staff lacked techniques to control the patients, the lobotomy gained popularity. Imagine, over 3,000 people living in a constant, nightmarish daze of insanity with no way to combat the horror of their illness. The anguish, terror, and utter hopelessness must have been an unbearable cross to bear, and its imprint has soaked into the walls and floors of the Weston State Hospital.

Perhaps the most tragic place is the children's wing, an area where orphans and unwanted children were placed because they had no parents or because their parents could no longer afford to keep them. But just because they had separate wings for children and the seriously disturbed doesn't mean they were separate from each other. All patients were allowed to roam the hospital wings, and it was fairly common for psychotics to mingle with children. Women were separated from the men in different wings, but this was little consolation, as the children's wing was adjacent to the men's wing.

But significant overcrowding and the quick deterioration of the facility forced the closure of the Weston State Hospital in 1994. The closing was so devastating to the little hamlet of Weston that the local economy was wracked by a debilitating recession that it has yet to recover from.

But in 2007, Joe Jordan, an asbestos demolitionist, paid $1.5 million for the old Weston State Hospital in a public auction, a steal compared to what he received in returned. Renaming it the Trans-Allegheny Lunatic Asylum, Jordan began to renovate the crumbling building and thus, re-invigorated the waning economy of Weston, West Virginia in the process.

Jacob and the Civil War Wing

The "Civil War Wing" is called that because it first admitted patients that had returned to their families from the bloody American Civil War in such states of madness that conventional therapies could not be applied. Shellshock and many other different forms of psychosis, as well as physical impairments such as tuberculosis were common ailments. It was also the very first in a series of wings that would make up the expansive and twisted hallways of Weston State Hospital.

Visitors to this area of the hospital have heard coughing, male laughter, and some have even been threatened with bodily harm should they not vacate the building immediately. But the most famous story involves the spirit of Jacob, a Civil War soldier who remains in the hospital to this day, roaming the halls and grounds as he would have done over 200 years before. Jacob's life and death are mysteries, and the common appearance of his ghost in and around the Civil War building is just as mysterious. His interest does not come easily, but women seem to be triggers for his attention, reacting as any soldier might to the presence of sweet-smelling, pretty girls, a welcome diversion to the suffering and foulness of his everyday life.

Today, most tour guides at the asylum refuse to enter the Civil War wing alone or at night, having reported being chased by the quick footsteps of a man who cannot be seen. They also report intense feelings of being watched, an unsettling feeling from unsettled spirits.

The Spirits of the Wards

The Trans-Allegheny Lunatic Asylum, being a Kirkbride-style building, is made up of different wards to facilitate the treatment of different types of patients. Up on the third floor, Ward C and Ward F held the more physically violent women and men, with only a single locked door separating the two wards. Tour guides in Ward F have reported being tapped on the shoulders, hearing the residual sounds of gurneys in the hallways, and sinister male voices whispering in their ears.

In Ward 2 on the second floor, victims of a double suicide and a particularly nasty stabbing have been known to frequent the dank hallways, their footsteps heard very clearly throughout the entire ward. A chilling brush of cold that seeps into your bones accompanies their footsteps and a pall seems to fall over the hallways until the footsteps, finally, dissipate into nothing and are gone.

It is in Ward 1 on the first floor that the Trans-Allegheny Lunatic Asylum's most cantankerous ghost resides. Her name was Ruth, and for many years, she called Ward C home. When the violent women of Ward C became too much for the frail and elderly Ruth, she was transferred to Ward 1, where she continued to claw and spout obscenities at passing orderlies and visitors. Her unruliness became such an issue that she spent much of her time strapped into a wheelchair, her hands fastened tightly to the wheelchair arms, mouth spewing curse words like Pez. When she died, it's believed that her spirit began to smack and push people, likely because no one could hear her taunts anymore.

When I visited the asylum in 2012, I was standing outside the doorway to Ward C and heard the horrific, bloodcurdling scream of an old woman, muffled, as if behind some locked door. I couldn't tell where it was coming from. It seemed to be from everywhere. No one else in the group but me and a young boy seemed to hear it; I automatically thought of Ruth and her clawing hands. But in a hospital where terror was a way of life, the screams of the damned could have belonged to anyone.

The Fourth Floor

Even while Trans-Allegheny was still in commission, there were stories of how haunted the fourth floor of the hospital actually was. The sounds of banging, footsteps, eerie laughter, and haunting screams echoed throughout. It is reputed to be such a haunted place that not even employees would willingly trek up to the fourth floor without an escort.

"I've seen it before, and I've heard it before," says Sue Parker, who was employed at Trans-Allegheny for thirty years as a psychiatric aide. "I knew that the fourth floor was haunted because I used to have to go up there after medical records. I could hear them following me."

Indeed, the sound of heavy footsteps following behind you are chilling, but what about the sounds of distant crying, screaming, and moaning? All of these symptoms point to that of a Residual Haunting. But paranormal investigators probing the fourth floor have collected EVPs of spirits answering specific questions as well as ordering them to "get out." Doors opening and closing on their own, strange sounds of banging, and even the muted sound of a conversation between two people have all been heard. Hospital gurneys have been known to have been spotted rolling down the hallways with no one behind them pushing.

The reports of meandering phantoms are also common, as is the case with many of the tour guides conducting their tours throughout the hospital. On numerous occasions, many different guides have reported seeing what they've thought was a man or a woman wandering the empty hallways. Thinking they were tourists lost within the building, the guides would go to check on them, and find nothing.

Also haunting the fourth floor is that of the spirit of a nurse, murdered by a patient who hid her body in an unused stairwell for nearly two months before she was found.

The Electroshock Therapy Rroom and the Morgue are also hotbeds of activity, with reports of screams and the sounds of invisible gurneys being pushed up and down the hallways. The full-bodied apparitions of both patients and doctors have been seen coming in and out of the rooms and roaming the desolate hallways, still on their rounds, or following their earthly routines.

Suicides, murder, and the natural deaths brought on by infections and disease claimed the lives of a huge number of people that quickly ballooned into the thousands during Trans-Allegheny's 136 years in operation. It should come as little to no surprise that the asylum has recently been named one of the most haunted in America.

Lilly

But the most famous ghost story of them all seems to be the tale of Lilly, the ghost of a three- or four-year-old girl who wanders the halls of Trans-Allegheny in search of her mother. Lilly's ghost has been particularly active when asked to play, as would be expected from a child, spirit or not.

Where did she come from? No one knows, though it is fairly certain that Lilly probably had been abandoned by her mother at the asylum and lived there for a few years before most likely succumbing to pneumonia or tuberculosis, common yet fatal childhood illnesses. Tales tell of her mother being a patient at Weston State Hospital, and that Lilly was born during her mother's incarceration. This story is widely popular, but lacks a realistic edge. Had Lilly's mother given birth to her while in Weston State Hospital, it is almost certain that Lilly would have been given over to an orphanage or adopted. Yet, there was a children's wing in Weston State Hospital, so it is possible that she endured there.

Today, it is believed that Lilly wanders the halls of Trans-Allegheny, seeking out the mother who had abandoned her so many years before, intent on finding her, yet not so serious about it that she will pass up playtime. Candy and plastic balls that have been left for Lilly have been found in places other than where they had been left, and investigators setting up in Lilly's room have heard giggling and small footsteps. Some tour guides and investigators have claimed to have played ball with Lilly, rolling a simple playground ball down the hallway, only to have it returned to them by some unseen force.

Lilly's story actually has the markings of the most basic of urban legends and there is a fairly large amount of skepticism attached to it as well. Perhaps it is just part of a legend that continues to grow amidst the horrible tales already swirling about this haunted place of suffering. Whether or not any of it is true, there is little doubt that this little soul is real and still calls the Weston State Hospital home.

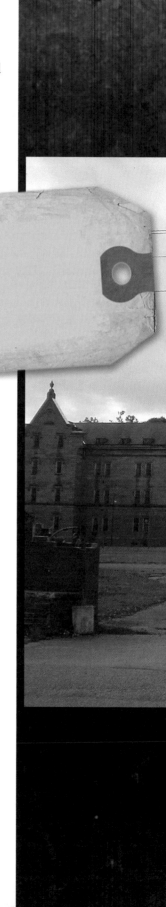

The Trans-Allegheny Lunatic Asylum

71 Asylum Drive
Weston, WV 26452
(304) 269-5070

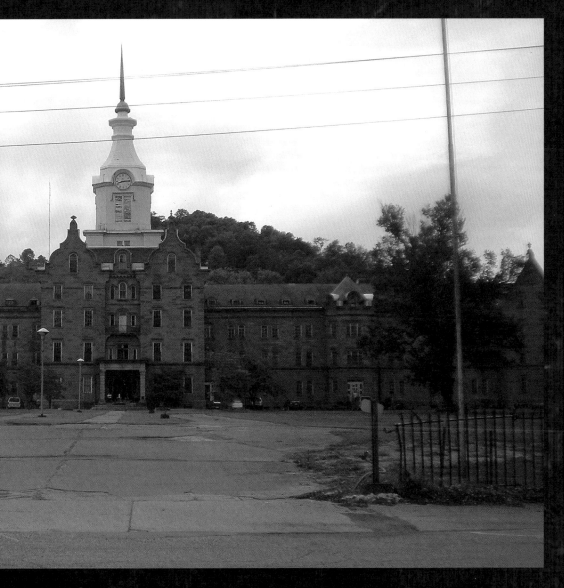

PHOTO 98 - PHOTO TRANS ALLEGHENY -EXT
The Trans-Allegheny Lunatic Asylum. *Photo courtesy of the author.*

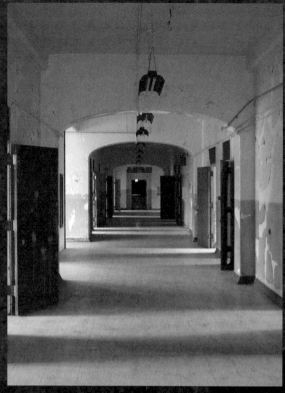

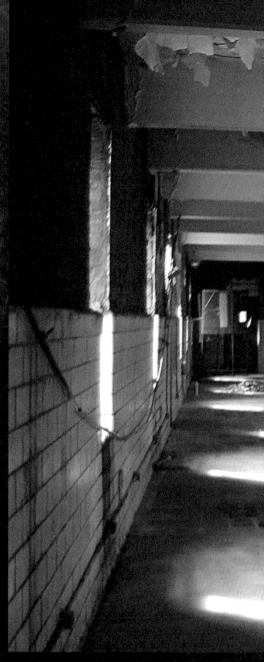

PHOTO 92 - TRANS ALLEGHENY 028
**Ward C of Trans-Allegheny, home of the more
violent female offenders.** *Photo courtesy of the author.*

PHOTO 96 - TRANS ALLEGHENY 017
The Civil War wing, the first building constructed and site of the first recorded haunting, that of

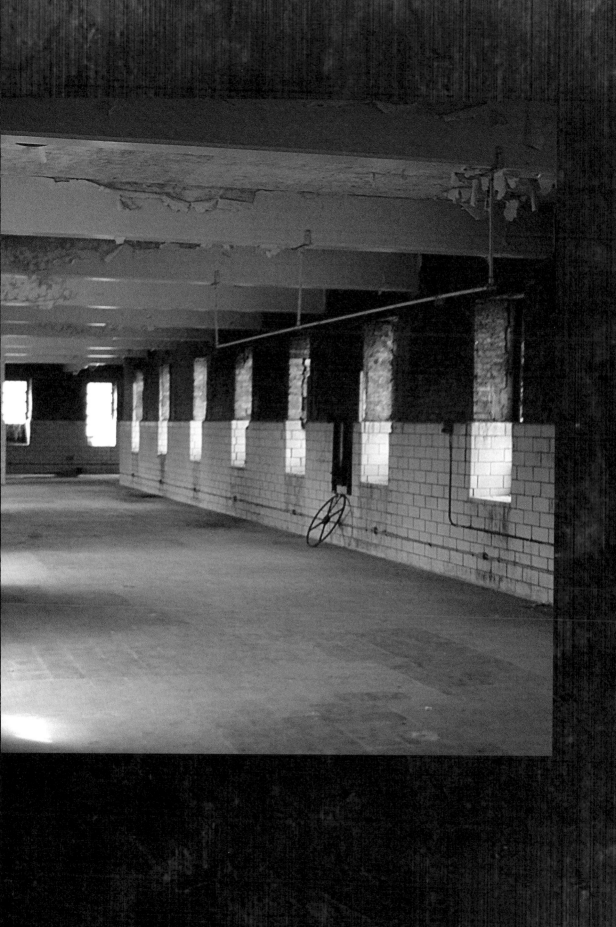

16.

LINDA VISTA COMMUNITY HOSPITAL
East Los Angeles, California
1904-1990

"I'm not afraid of werewolves or vampires or haunted hotels, I'm afraid of what real human beings do to other real human beings."

~Walter Jon Williams

Linda Vista Community Hospital shares a great number of similarities with the Ancora Psychiatric Hospital—the most notable being the number of people who disbelieve in the supposed hauntings within. Its reputation as a haunted hospital was brought to the mass audiences with the infamous *Ghost Adventures* episode in which Zak, Nick, and Aaron investigated and received some interesting evidence. But before *Ghost Adventures* even aired the episode, Linda Vista Community Hospital was considered one of the most prolifically haunted spots in Los Angeles by many people in the Southern California paranormal circles.

Located in the East Los Angeles suburb called Boyle Heights, Linda Vista began life in 1904 as a hospital for nearby railroad workers. Situated across the street from Hollenbeck Park, it exclusively treated and rehabilitated workers of the Sante Fe Railroad Company. A simple, yet well-planned building, reconstruction began in 1925 for what would become the building we see today. It was a happy place with bright-colored rooms and a cheerful demeanor. Mexican migrants were segregated from the white and black patients, but all received equal care that was unparalleled at the time.

As the hospital flourished, additional wings were built onto the existing main building, including more floors for patients and their recreational pursuits. But in 1937, the railroad abdicated ownership of the hospital and it reopened to the public that same year as the Linda Vista Community Hospital.

Some say that this is when the reputation and care of Linda Vista Hospital began to take a darker turn for the worse. Over the years, the care and optimism, traits that had long defined Linda Vista, had begun to wane. Railroad money was slowly replaced with anemic funding from the state of California, and many of the features that defined Linda Vista as one of the premier hospitals of Los Angeles simply disappeared; lack of funding led to a drop in quality employment.

By the time the mid-1980s were in full swing, Linda Vista found itself in the middle of war-torn South Central Los Angeles. As a result, the emergency room saw more than its fair share of gunshot and stabbing victims of all ages and races. Most had no insurance. Steadily, good doctors began to leave Linda Vista for higher paying jobs in safer environments. By 1988, Linda Vista had begun to refuse ambulance services, working exclusively on people who walked in off the streets. To top it all off, the rumors (founded and unfounded) of patient abuse at the hands of the staff led to cuts in funding.

In 1990, as the hospital administration faced multiple malpractice lawsuits and incredible budget cuts from the California government, it was decided that the hospital should close. Since the closing, it has become a highly sought after location for film productions, namely *In The Line Of Fire, Pearl Harbor, End Of Days, Outbreak,* and, most famously, as the original hospital in the pilot episode of *ER*.

Rumor has it that the hospital was abandoned so quickly that personal files, surgical instruments, medical supplies, and furniture still dot the interior's landscape. It is possible that these implements were left behind by film productions, but the pounds of human ash in the basement crematory speak another story, one that could not be made up. Presumably filled with the ashes of unclaimed John and Jane Does, the ash catch tray now acts as a steel tomb for what could be multiple bodies.

As film and television productions continued to use Linda Vista Hospital as a set for their dramas, more stories of peculiar and frightening things began to circulate. Screams and moans were heard by more than a few actors and production associates. Darting shadows, flickering lights, faded green lights, and a foul odor emanating from the third floor are all red flags that seem to point to signs of a haunting.

But it isn't just these classic tell-tale signals of hauntings that make people believe. For some, the sight of a ghostly doctor wearing a tie, as he looks out a corner window is enough. He stands there stoically, gazing off into some distant future before disappearing from view.

Roaming the third-floor hallways is the spirit of a young woman who paces the cold linoleum floors aimlessly. Recent paranormal investigations have recorded EVPs of the spirit announcing her name as "Chloe." Interestingly enough, this spirit seems to have a special connection to another spirit: that of a little girl killed in a car accident in front of the hospital in the early 1990s. Chloe seems very protective of the young child, who makes herself known with innocent, yet thoroughly chilling, giggles. Anyone attempting to contact the little girl often finds their way blocked by Chloe, whose fierce determination protects the girl from strangers. I find this incredibly inspiring and pretty darn unnerving. Personally speaking, I wish more spirits like Chloe were out there protecting the young, even after death.

In addition to Chloe and the young girl, witnesses say another spirit wanders the desolate property: that of a former doctor. A search for the identity of this spirit points to a man named Dr. Edwards, who was murdered on the property in the mid-1980s. He was an ER doctor who treated the leader of a notorious gang for a nasty series of bullet wounds incurred in a drive-by shooting. While he did all that he could, it was not nearly enough, and the gang leader eventually succumbed to his wounds. When his followers found out, they not only tracked down and killed the shooters, but also found Dr. Edwards and shot him to death, execution style, in the parking lot as he walked to his car.

On the top floor of the hospital in a corner office window, bystanders and investigators alike have seen the apparition of this doctor, dressed nicely in a blue tie and white coat. He stands at the window, looking out over Boyle Heights, only to slowly disappear from view. This same doctor has been seen walking through the hospital's dark corridors, a Residual Haunting that shows him still doing his rounds.

Outside of Linda Vista—directly next door, I might add—is a building that has been repeatedly, and erroneously, identified as the Psychiatric Ward. It is, in fact, the Nurse's Dormitory, a building used to house the various nurses, nurses' assistants, and volunteers. A small network of tunnels underneath both buildings connected them together and made it easier for the nurses to travel back and forth from building to building. But it is in the Dormitory where they say a demonic influence targets women, pushing, pulling, and groping them inside various rooms on all floors. Terrifying attacks, scratches, and devilish voices have been recorded by varying investigative teams. It is difficult to say how, where, and why this demonic influence came about, but given that the building was prone to trespassers and paranormal groups alike, any number of portals could have been opened inside Linda Vista—opened and never closed.

It is all of these things that made Linda Vista Hospital stand out in the paranormal community, a swirling vortex of paranormal activity that is matched only by Waverly Hills.

Or is it?

A casual debate exists between those who believe and those who find the idea of Linda Vista being haunted ludicrous. Some employees have come forward with their paranormal experiences, and some have come forward discounting the hauntings. However, in the opinions of numerous paranormal investigation teams and the massive amounts of unexplained evidence they have collected, it would seem that Linda Vista *is* haunted, for after the lights go down and the silence reclaims the hallways, the voices and actions of the past are heard, felt, and seen.

Linda Vista Community Hospital

610 Saint Louis Street
Los Angeles, CA 90023

It is privately owned and trespassers will be arrested.

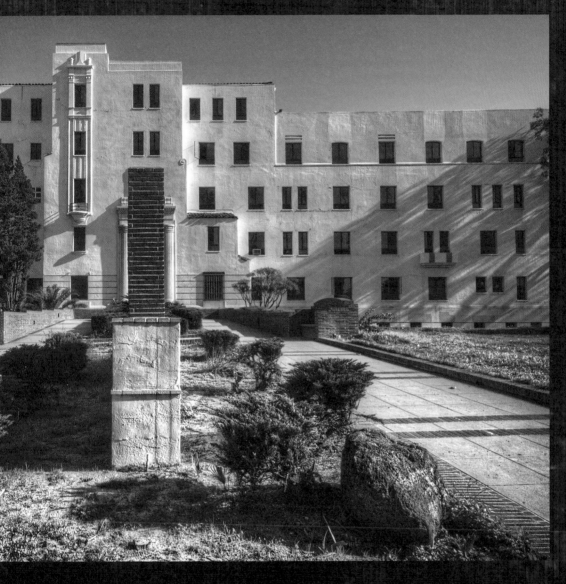

Linda Vista Community Hospital. *Photo courtesy of Neil Kremer, Creative Commons License.*

17.

OLD IDAHO STATE PENITENTIARY
Boise, Idaho
1872-1973

"There is a close relationship between flowers and convicts. The fragility and delicacy of the former are of the same nature as the brutal insensitivity of the latter."

~Jean Genet

Every state has one. In fact, I believe that nearly every city, 'burg, and town in the United States has one. It is almost a guarantee that everyone reading this right now remembers their hometown boogeyman, a scary guy who committed an awful crime and paid for it in just as awful a way. Or worse, was never caught and made to pay penance for it. The people of Los Angeles feared the "Black Dahlia Killer." Those in Fall River, Massachusetts locked their doors to keep Lizzie Borden from axing them to death. For the people of Idaho, their boogeyman came in the form of Raymond Allan Snowden, a merciless killer who brutally murdered pretty Cora Dean on September 23, 1956. His execution at Boise's Idaho State Penitentiary was equally horrific, yet most witnesses barely flinched.

Opened in 1872, Idaho's State Penitentiary was a Romanesque masterpiece of confinement. Its twenty-foot-high walls made it nearly impossible for people on the outside to see in, and it made it unbearable for prisoners longing to see the outside world. Like Eastern State Penitentiary in Pennsylvania, the architects of Idaho's penitentiary emphasized isolation and a marked removal of the convicts from anything remotely related to the outside world.

Any executions ordered in the state of Idaho were carried out at the Old Idaho State Penitentiary in the open-air gallows just outside the main cell blocks, but still within the prison walls; apparently, families would gather on nearby hilltops to watch the hangings.

Like all prisons, the Old Idaho State Penitentiary was home to a lot of bad people and a lot of bad things happened, but nothing in my research compares to the story of what happened in the showers to one unfortunate inmate who entered intent on getting cleaned up, only to find himself the main character in one of the most gruesome attacks I have ever researched. Unfortunately, his name has been lost to the ages, but after you hear what happened to him, his ghost and his family might appreciate the anonymity.

Allegedly occurring in the late 1960s, this prisoner was cornered in the shower room by five men who had taken exception to his conviction of being a multiple child molester and a rather prolific pedophile at that. In this shower room, the prisoner was gang raped, the attack so brutal and so overpowering that his body eventually gave out and he died on the shower floor in a heap of blood and mangled, manhandled flesh. No one was ever brought to trial for it and it is thought that because the attack lasted so long and the screams of the dying man were so loud that guards at the penitentiary must have been looking the other way while it was happening.

Of course, there will be some who say that it was a justified murder; pedophiles get what they deserve and the punishment doled out by the courts is nothing compared to the punishments fellow convicts dish out. But no one can deny the shocking power of that terrifying act and the horror that must have been left behind in its wake. To this day, there is speculation that not only does the ghost of the murdered pedophile still haunt the shower room, but the ghosts of his attackers stalk the shower room as well. Black, fleeting shadows have been seen darting about on occasion and the residual screams of the dying man have been caught once or twice by vigilant ghost hunters staking out the place.

In the prison courtyard, where a rose garden now sits, is where the gallows used to be set up. This patch of land saw an incredible amount of death, yet it is the ghost of the inmate groundskeeper who appears, having been spotted by tourists tending to the rose garden that replaced the gallows scaffold.

Raymond Allan Snowden

As I mentioned before, for a long time and to many older residents of Idaho, the resident boogeyman was a murderer named Raymond Allan Snowden. Before September 23, 1956, Snowden was a mere petty criminal, doing time for burglary here, a stint for petty theft there. But on the night of the 23rd, he became Idaho's most famous murderer. In the town of Garden City, pretty 48-year-old Cora Lucyle Dean had met Snowden at a club called the HiHo. Dean was a recent divorcee, still reeling from the desertion of her husband when she fell for the rapt attention Snowden paid to her. After some dances, it was reported that they left together. When Snowden refused to pay for a cab to take her back to Boise, an argument ensued, wherein Cora began to hit and knee Snowden.

"She swung and at the same time she kneed me again," said Snowden in his confession to police. "I blew my top." It was in this moment that Snowden gave Cora Dean an ultimatum: "Rape or death! It's your choice, honey!"

Cora Dean quickly made her decision, kicking Snowden in the crotch.

In a fit of rage, Snowden attacked Cora Dean and cut her throat with a three-inch bone-handled pocket knife. He then used the knife to stab her corpse over thirty times, the attack culminating in Snowden severing her spinal cord with the blade. He left her lying in the driveway of a paint factory, where she would be found sometime later that night.

Fleeing the murder, Snowden sought refuge in Hannifen's Cigar Store in nearby Boise, ditching the knife in the gutter outside where it was later recovered by police. The clerk on duty remembered Snowden entering the store, looking disheveled, his hands bloody. He made his way to the bathroom and cleaned up, exiting quickly afterward.

Detectives closed in on Snowden when a former girlfriend came forward and said that Snowden had threatened to sever her spinal cord. This, combined with the eyewitness testimony of the cigar store clerk, proved enough to arrest Raymond Allan Snowden for the murder of Cora Dean. Because of the pure and unadulterated ferocity of the murder, a detective magazine at the time dubbed Snowden "Idaho's Jack The Ripper."

Not surprisingly, Snowden was convicted of the murder and sentenced to hang at the Old Idaho Penitentiary. During the course of his initial incarceration, Snowden also confessed to the murders of two other women, but a lack of evidence prevented authorities from prosecuting him.

On October 18, 1957, a little over a year since he'd murdered Cora Dean, Snowden was executed in the gallows room of the Idaho Penitentiary. But the hangman's mistake of not tying the noose correctly made Snowden's execution almost unwatchable. For fifteen minutes, Snowden hung from his neck, strangling slowly before finally succumbing to the rope. His execution was the last one performed at the Old Idaho State Penitentiary, and another execution would not be performed again until 1994.

What makes Snowden's case so interesting to paranormal investigators is the fact that his ghost haunts in both an intelligent and a residual way. In the 5 House of the Old Idaho State Penitentiary, his presence has been made known by banging noises, light touches, and the occasional EVP of a male voice. His shade has been seen inside the cell he occupied while awaiting the hangman, the dark misty apparition foreshadowing its appearance with blasts of cold air and bolts of highly charged static electricity that raise the hair on your neck and arms.

Additionally, Snowden's spirit makes an appearance at Hannifan's Cigar Store, entering as he did in 1956, using the restroom, and exiting the store, all classic markings of a Residual Haunting. It could be confusing if one didn't make the distinction between Residual and Intelligent Hauntings; after all, how could one ghost be in two places at once? But the ramifications of his crime obviously have left quite an imprint on the fabric of time and space in the normally quiet state of Idaho, for his ghost is still reported to show itself on occasion, performing the same way he did in 1956, without deviation in the slightest.

Old Idaho State Penitentiary
2445 Old Penitentiary Road
Boise, ID 83712

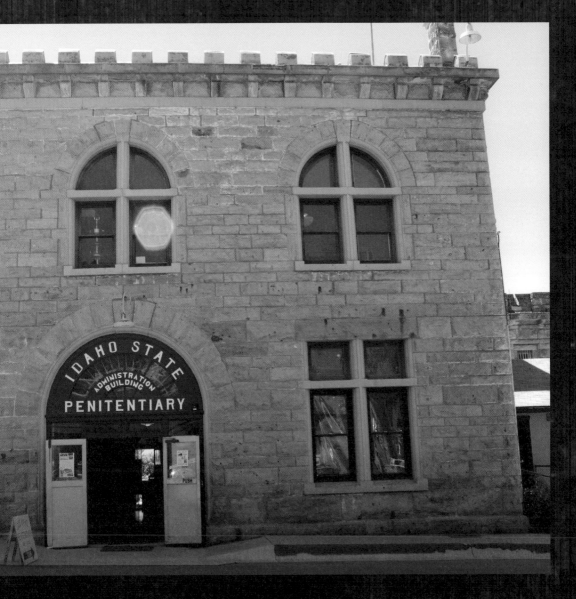

PHOTO: 42 - IDAHO STATE PEN EXTERIOR
Photo courtesy of Salle Neate.

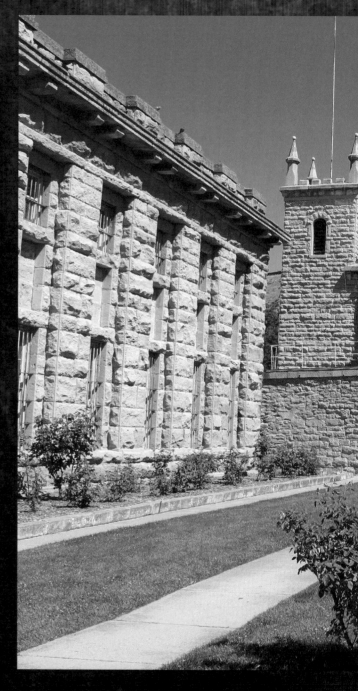

PHOTO 40 - IDAHO STATE PEN GALLOWS AREA
There is a rose and flower garden here now, but in 1872, this was the original spot used for the gallows. *Photo courtesy of Salle Neate.*

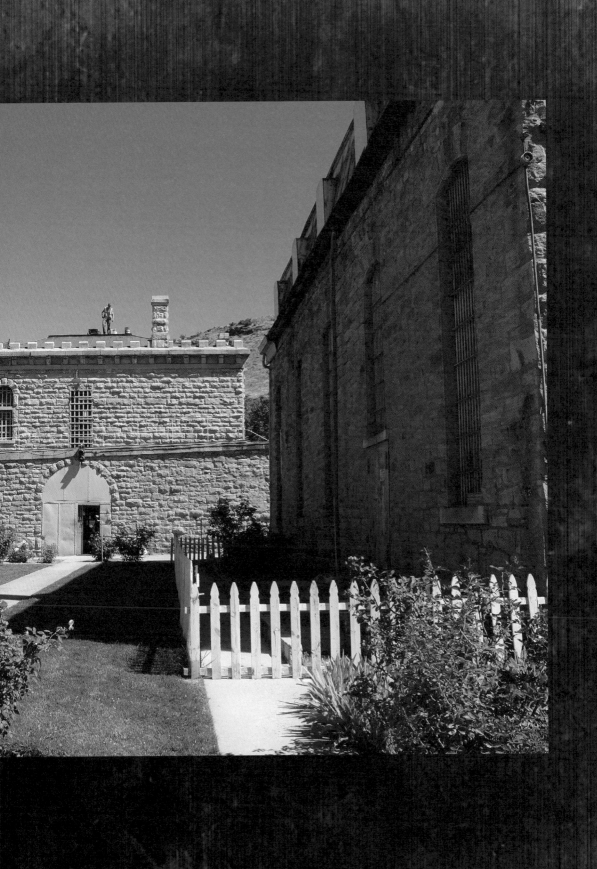

18.

NORWICH STATE HOSPITAL

Preston, Connecticut

1904-1996

"A casual stroll through the lunatic asylum shows that faith does not prove anything."
~Friedrich Nietzsche

It is simply one of those buildings that needs no introduction. Like Danvers, Central State, and the Trans-Allegheny Lunatic Asylum, Norwich State Hospital sits high on the list of ghost hunters' paradise and is routinely referred to simply as Norwich. Built in 1904, Norwich opened its doors for the mentally unhinged, the chemically dependent, the mentally retarded, and the criminally insane. Quite a laundry list of psychoses, indeed, and one that Norwich seems to embrace. A place like the Norwich State Hospital is one of the reasons paranormal investigators refer to Connecticut as the most haunted state in the Union.

Norwich State initially sat on just about a hundred acres; over the years, more land was developed and 300 acres was added to the property. Today, Norwich State houses over thirty buildings, each with a different purpose, from a machine shop to the patient dormitories, to the Inebriate Farm and a clubhouse for employees. All of these buildings sprung up over a period of some fifty years, erected as patient population grew.

In 1904, they initially treated only 95 patients. But by 1950, they were housing and rehabilitating well over 3,000. A tremendous spike in the population was felt in the 1930s when the massive tuberculosis outbreak struck much of the United States and Norwich adapted its policies and practices to include the treatment of these unfortunate tubercular patients.

Of particular interest is the setting of the hospital. For years, paranormal researchers have hypothesized that bodies of water, such as rivers or lakes, can intensify spiritual energy, making a spirit more likely to manifest in some physical way, whether it be through EVPs, apparitions, or the physical manipulation of the world around them: places like Bobby Mackey's in Wilder, Kentucky, which neighbors the Licking River, and the Trans-Allegheny Lunatic Asylum in Weston, West Virginia, which calls the west fork of the Monongahela River a neighbor.

Norwich State is no exception: its front door overlooks the Thames River.

In 1914, the first documented instance of suicide was reported when a male patient hung himself in the bathrooms of his particular ward. From then on, it seemed that a death curse had begun to circulate about Norwich. Two employees died from wounds they sustained when a water heater exploded. Additionally, a nurse eventually took her own life after returning home from a particularly taxing shift at the hospital.

In 1939, a rather nasty outbreak of dysentery began to run rampant through the Women's Ward of Norwich. Nurses, doctors, and other members of the staff tried frantically to find and isolate the cause of the outbreak, but the lives of fourteen elderly women came to an abrupt and painful end before it was contained. This outbreak was met head on by another in 1947, this time as a deadly strain of influenza claimed the lives of sixty people. The accepted reason: a shortage of nurses and staff made it impossible to treat everyone. To those living at Norwich, life was a waking nightmare. To those on the outside, it was a dark, bloated monster who struck fear into the hearts of all who stared into its darkness. It was the extreme version of a cautionary tale. Of particular note is the spectrum of ages that called Norwich home.

Eleven-year-old Robert Curgenven was sentenced to Norwich for the shooting deaths of his parents and his younger brother in 1956. His reasoning? His parents had spanked him, and his younger brother constantly picked on him. Doctors diagnosed him as a massive paranoid schizophrenic and he spent the rest of his days behind the walls of Norwich.

Like Curgenven, 15-year-old Paul Babcock, who had been sentenced to Norwich for the attack on a young girl two years earlier, was charged with the bludgeoning murder of a 7-year-old fellow patient at Norwich named Richard Otis.

Twenty-five-year-old sexual serial killer Michael B. Ross made Norwich's dark history in 1983 when he raped and murdered a 19-year-old girl in the woods surrounding the hospital. In the end, he was convicted of murdering six women in the state of Connecticut and handed multiple life sentences after he confessed to avoid the death penalty.

Fires, an uncommonly high number of suicides, murders, rapes, and random acts of general mayhem, helped to solidify Norwich's reputation as a genuinely frightening place to be. This is just a drop in the bucket compared to the real life horror that happened regularly at Norwich and numerous other mental institutions' campuses. That thick, dense atmosphere of pain, horror, terror, and sadness hangs heavy in places like this and nothing can make it go away easily.

But still, in the midst of all this horror, the medical workers, doctors, and nurses still tried their very best to care for their patients. Most workers, who made very little money themselves, went out of their way to buy Christmas gifts for every patient in their wards, and every Halloween was met with decorations and in-hospital Trick-or-Treating.

"It wasn't all 'Cuckoo's Nest'," says Steven DePolito, a documentary filmmaker whose father worked in the kitchens of Norwich. "Amazing things did happen, that sense of family. It wasn't the haunted asylum. I want people to understand that people there did the best they could with what they had in a very difficult job."

The hospital closed in 1996 and the remaining 1,000 or so patients were transferred to the nearby Connecticut Valley Hospital. There was talk of demolition, which gave rise to ideas of amusement parks, playgrounds, and museums dedicated to the suffering of the mentally damaged, but as of yet, none have been taken so seriously.

Norwich State Hospital, crippled, abandoned, and rotting, still stands, and to this day, still houses the lonely souls of those patients so troubled that they cannot find their way out. So troubled in fact are these specters that they continually engage the trespassers upon their home in hostile and shocking ways. Objects have been thrown at people, tossed down long hallways and striking at precise points on the floor, or tagging investigators in the back. Clothes have been tugged, hands grabbed, and people have been shoved, all by unseen beings that seem to love trying to get attention and scare the hell out of visitors.

In surgical suites where lobotomies and torturous hydrotherapies had been performed, visitors and security guards have reported the residual sounds of hospital equipment "beeping" as if an EKG or breathing machine is still in use. Of course, there is no power in the building, let alone expensive medical equipment that could make such noises.

Urban explorers have often targeted Norwich State Hospital as a pristine example of a building ripe for exploration. But their adventurous attitudes have also been met by dark shadow figures, whispering voices in the dark, and the soft padding of footsteps that are not their own.

It is the tunnels, however—like the ones at Waverly Hills, Central State, and Rolling Hills Asylum—that seem to hold the most hostility at Norwich. High-risk prisoners, such as arsonists, murderers, and rapists, were chained to chairs in the tunnels and faced routine beatings by orderlies and nurses' aides. It is rumored that some doctors performed surgical and drug-induced experiments on these unfortunates as well, and that their ghosts haunt the tunnels running under the Salmon Building.

In other parts of the buildings, the very few paranormal groups granted permission to investigate at Norwich State have reported the murmurings of voices and whispers, recorded not only as EVPs, but as valid sounds heard by their own ears. Unnerving blankets of cold air have enveloped the warmest rooms, and the heartrending sounds of a woman weeping uncontrollably have also been heard echoing throughout the desolate hallways.

But it isn't always the audible voices that one hears in Norwich State. What frightens people the most about Norwich are the voices heard within your head as you traverse the crumbling corridors of this once stately and protective city unto itself. Multiple ghost hunters and skeptics alike have reported the unsettling feeling of hearing strange voices in their own minds, as if the spirits were communicating with the living through a form of extra sensory perception (ESP).

This hospital is a prime example that a haunted place doesn't need a traumatic history in order to be haunted. Norwich State Hospital proves that all you need for a good haunting is the very real emotional and mental traumas its thousands of patients have endured during their lives and continue to endure well into their deaths.

Psychic Impressions

Remote viewing of Norwich State Hospital left me out in the cold, so to speak. As I tried to hone in on some of the spirits dwelling within the old asylum, I found my way inside blocked by a thick wall of psychic energy, put there not by the spirits, but by the people of Preston, Connecticut. It is my belief that they have erected this wall of psychic energy subconsciously because they want to keep out any and all intruders who wish to try and exploit Norwich State's history.

One cannot blame them, not in the least. This is indeed an age of exploitation, but my goal has always been to see the human face behind the hauntings.

Refocusing my energy, I eased my way into the underground tunnels, passing by spirits of every age and sex. There was a lot of residual energy held inside the walls like a sponge holds onto water. It is likely that if this energy were dissipated and expelled, the buildings known as Norwich State Hospital would probably collapse in on itself.

There was one woman who stopped me in the tunnels, pushing me away with a hand. She wouldn't allow me to go any further. She told me, "It's not safe. You can't go any further." Her will was strong and I obeyed her wishes; there was a lightness in her eyes that seemed to make my resolve wilt. But before I left, I saw the darkness beyond her and realized how much of a favor she was doing for me.

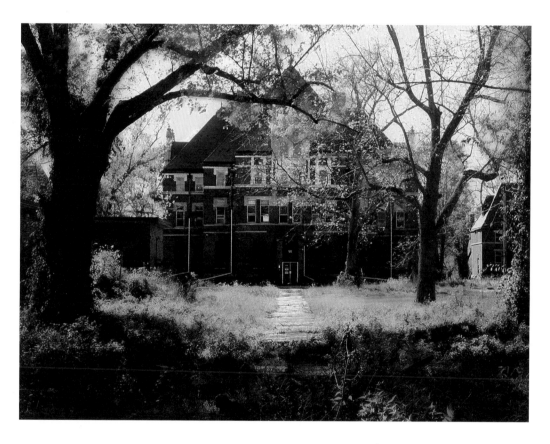

PHOTO 43 - NORWICH EXTERIOR
Norwich State Hospital. *Photo courtesy of Aimee Lindell.*

Norwich State Hospital is located in the town of Preston, Connecticut and is strictly off limits to the public. On-site security guards *will* call police and have you arrested for trespassing.

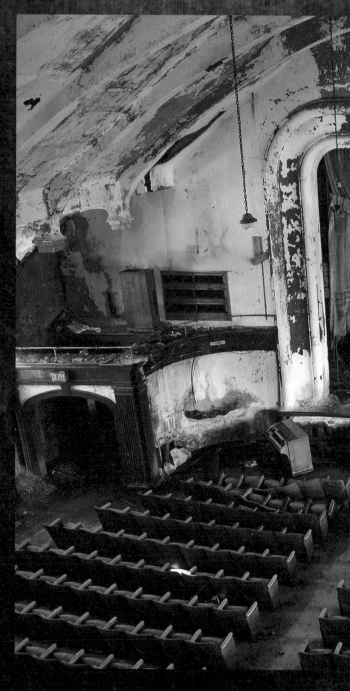

The auditorium of Norwich State Hospital. *Photo courtesy of Kevin Husta, Owl's Flight Photography.*

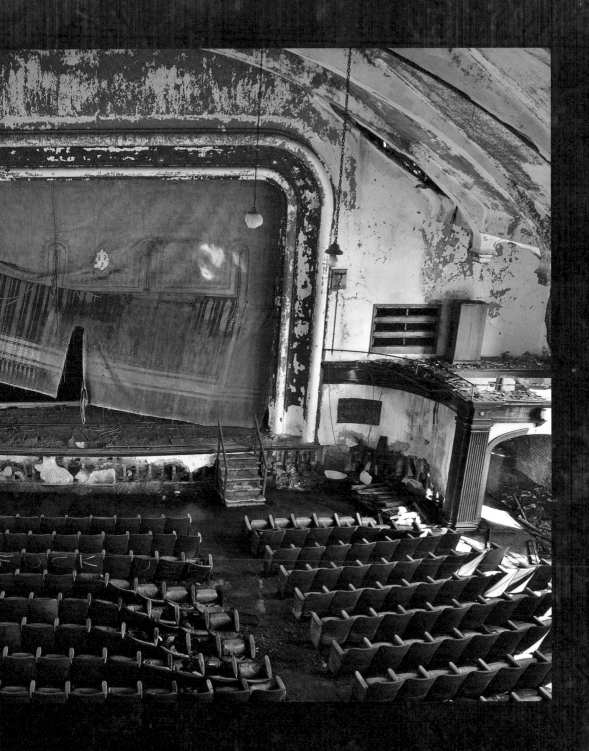

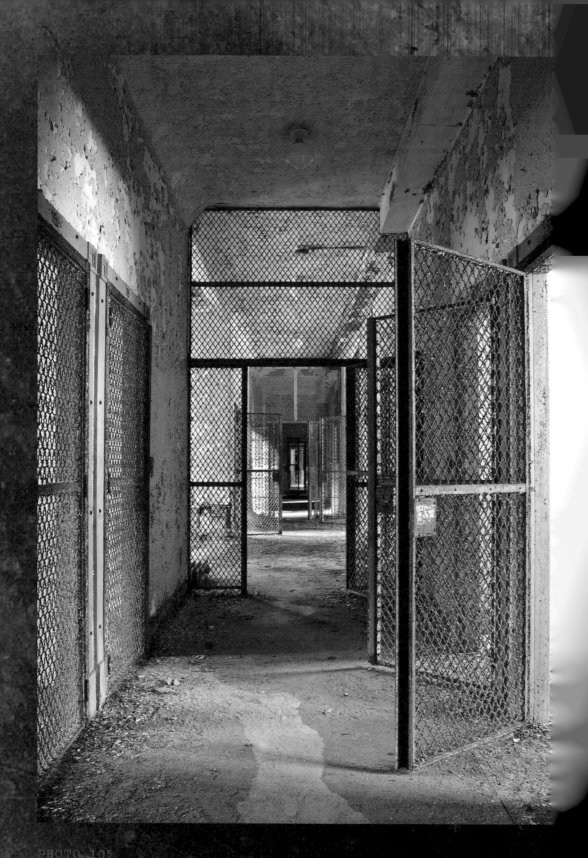

19.
CLOVIS AVENUE SANITARIUM
Clovis, California
1922-1997

"It is, alas, chiefly the evil emotions that are able to leave their photographs on surrounding scenes and objects and whoever heard of a place haunted by a noble deed, or of beautiful and lovely ghosts revisiting the glimpses of the moon?"

~Algernon H. Blackwood

Like many other mental health facilities, Clovis Avenue Sanitarium began with the best of intentions. In a world where the emotionally crippled and thoroughly deranged seemingly began to outnumber the sane, the opening of Clovis Avenue Sanitarium was a godsend. But somewhere, during its long history, the story took a dark turn and the legend of one of the world's most feared haunted places began.

The town of Clovis, California lies at the feet of the Sierra Nevadas, a perfect gateway to the mountainous region known for its coal, gold, and burgeoning petroleum ventures. It was here that Italian immigrant Tony Andriotti decided to build his dream home, an opulent mansion that would be his crowning glory. The initial structure was completed in 1922, but the shear cost of the project, aided by the Great Depression, put Andriotti into total bankruptcy. In 1935, alcoholic and emotionally desperate, Andriotti took his own life.

Initially, the house became a hospice of sorts for those with terminal illnesses, such as cancer and tuberculosis. At this time, it was called the Hazelwood Sanitarium. It is a safe bet that many patients, suffering beyond belief, breathed their last behind the walls of this opulent mansion. But after seven years, ownership changed once again. The house came into possession of a woman named Mrs. Brashears, who set out to convert the manor into a convalescent home for the mentally ill. To accommodate more patients, two separate additions were built onto the existing mansion, with each addition specializing in different types of behaviors. Opened officially in 1942, with the cooperation of the California government and the ability to house just over 150 people, the beds quickly began to fill up.

The terms and definitions of mental illness were especially broad in those days. From something as innocuous as homosexuality to the thoroughly demented madness of paranoid schizophrenia, it was all considered mental illness that needed hospitalization to treat. Everyone took advantage of these facts by committing their loved ones, considered burdens of the time, to their local insane asylums. Thus, it was no surprise that the population boomed well over the comfortable capacity of just 150. It has been said that there were so many patients at Clovis Sanitarium that every available space was taken with a bed. Six to seven cots were packed into each bedroom. Gurneys lined the hallways, the patients strapped down to keep them from moving. There were even incidents of patients being tied to shower pipes, toilets, and handrails. The high levels of anxiety brought out the worst in the patients and they often turned on each other, with deadly results.

Clovis Sanitarium was probably very understaffed, mostly due to the fact that the state of California would have only given enough money to the asylum to pay workers caring for 150 patients or less. With the overcrowding problem, one runs into the nightmarish predicament of possibly only two nurses for fifty people. Unfortunately, neglect and abuse became a sad, yet normal, practice. These people, even today, testify to the brutal conditions, neglect, abuse, and torture bestowed upon these unfortunates of the state.

One amenity that hadn't been planned, but probably should have been, was a morgue. Oddly, there hadn't even been an official morgue when Clovis Sanitarium had been Hazelwood Sanitarium, the hospital for the terminally ill. Until the corpses could be picked up by local authorities, the bodies would lie in the cool of the basement for undetermined lengths of time.

Finally, in 1997, Clovis Sanitarium was shut down, closed for good. After seventy-five years and countless deaths later, the legend of Clovis Sanitarium the Hospital became the legend of Clovis Sanitarium the Haunted. The haunted spirit of Tony Andriotti was now joined by the thousands of enraged, demented, and melancholy souls swallowed up by Clovis.

Stories of strange goings on at the former sanitarium swirled about the town, becoming notorious. But unlike most tales told around campfires, many of them were true. It began with the stories trespassers and vandals would tell their friends, tales about their hair getting pulled, the disturbing sounds of a walker being dragged across the floor, doors slamming shut on their own, and the shadows of former patients, both adult and child, darting about the inside.

The house on Clovis Avenue was now, officially, the scar of Clovis, California, an unfortunate blight that would not go away. People stopped talking about it. Children crossed the street to avoid walking on its sidewalk. It was Clovis' elephant in the room, a place that reminded them daily of the abuse and horror that once went on behind those old walls.

A bona fide skeptic, Todd Wolfe, purchased the old house in 2008, with hopes of turning it into a haunted attraction he would call "Scream If You Can." His skepticism was immediately put to rest when he felt hot breath on the back of his neck and spun around to find no one there. This was only the beginning of his experiences. Clovis Wolfe Manor, as he had re-christened it, was haunted beyond belief. He had the hospital wing behind the mansion demolished soon after he purchased the estate and allegedly allowed a psychic to coax several harmless entities that haunted the rubble to come and find haven in the mansion.

This is what is called "opening a doorway." When the psychic coaxed these two seemingly harmless entities into the mansion itself, he or she had to open a psychic doorway that made such a thing possible. Unfortunately, when a psychic doorway is opened and never properly closed, any kind of spiritual energy, good or bad, can walk in.

That is perhaps why Clovis Wolfe Manor is so haunted. Not only are there the violent spirits of its former residents haunting the place, but also the possibly very dark entities that were allowed in when the portal was opened and, very likely, never closed.

Dark entities are, for lack of a better term, cannibals that feed on the energy of lesser spirits and those living souls brave enough to trudge through the location.

In any case, this was something Todd Wolfe was now banking on. Even today, by going to their website, you can sign up to view their Ghost Cams, and Todd Wolfe and his colleagues host regular ghost hunts that are streamed live on the Internet.

Perhaps the strangest of incidents ever recorded by someone, other than paranormal investigators, involve the occurrence of chilling calls to 911 from someone inside the house on Clovis Avenue. Clovis police were often dispatched to the old asylum, responding to mysterious 911 calls that were said to originate from inside the house. But the absence of a working phone line, as well as electricity, created more questions than answers. When 911 dispatchers received the calls, they heard only dead air—an ominous, static hum on the other end. So who was calling 911? And more importantly, what did they want?

But before we let the shivers take control of our reason, let's remember that Clovis Wolfe Manor was once a hospital, a clinic, and an insane asylum, and because of that, the hospital was most likely outfitted with a security system that would ring the police in the case of an emergency. During power outages and blackouts, it is entirely possible that this security system would automatically dial the police as a precaution. With the power disabled to Clovis Wolfe Manor, but not the security system, it is possible that the security system misinterpreted the power outage as an emergency and kept calling the police on its own. This was a theory that was eventually brought up on the *Ghost Hunters* television show, but it in no way debunks the myriad other paranormal occurrences that happen there on a regular basis.

As we've learned before, spirits are not without their intelligence or their passion. Isn't is possible that a spirit, which is made up entirely of energy, has learned how to manipulate the system and call for the help he or she has been calling out for years?

The Man Babies

One of the oddest tales to come from Clovis Wolfe Manor is the tales of the so-called Man Baby ghosts. Several investigators, including paranormal investigators and EVP experts Mark and Debby Constantino, have had run-ins with pint-sized spirits that resemble children in appearance, but have the faces of grown men. Their skin is said to be beige and rubbery and they never seem to be wearing clothes. They are sometimes accompanied by Shadow People and seem to want to interact with the living, but their outward appearance tends to alienate those who are lucky enough to catch sight of them, mostly because it is hard to separate the mannish face from the baby body. They're just an odd, weird sight to behold.

The Man Babies have also been seen on the first floor, in the sunroom, and in the attic crawlspace.

So what are these mysterious Man Babies? Some parapsychologists believe that they seem to be darker spirits who feed off of emotions: good, bad, or indifferent. If the emotional state of the living or the dead is heightened and at an apex, these so-called Man Babies consider that to be dinner time. Their only purpose is to feed on charged-up, energy-laden emotions and psychic energy. Are they demonic, or just plain parasitical spirits who use the image of a child to get what they want?

Mary and George's Room

The identity of "Mary" is not certain, but the room occupied by her spirit is one of the more famous—and infamous—haunts in the whole house. She is a timid old lady, it is said, who likes to sing. Rumor has it that the room used to be a surgical suite while the house was opened as a hospice for terminally ill patients, and Mary just may have been one of those patients who lost her life on the operating table. Her spirit is said to be one of the more harmless shades within the house, and when she is near, the temperature drops significantly and EVPs of an older woman begin to come through on many investigators' digital recorders.

Even more interesting is the idea that, should you move one of the chairs in the room, Mary will move it back to its rightful place.

Just down the way from Mary's room is George's room. But in this case, the identity of George has been validated; former nurses claim that a cantankerous old man named George once occupied the room in question. Furthermore, EVPs have been captured of an old man saying the name "George" repeatedly, backing up the nurses' stories in chilling detail. Being a popular name, "George" could be any number of patients or retirees who once called the sanitarium home in its long history, however.

In this room, most people feel the negative presence of a woman, but know that George is there as well. While no clear paranormal activity has been reported in this room, it is still a compelling companion to Mary's room, with fairly clear EVPs being documented from within.

The Basement

In many instances of haunted places, there is a battle of wills between the good and the dark spirits, all vying for control of the spiritual realm in which they live. But at Clovis Wolfe Manor, the division between the light and the dark has never been more clear or more defined. It is here, in the bowels of Clovis Wolfe Manor, that the darkest entities seem to reside, feeding on the dark energy left behind by the dead and dying. Just as the more benign spirits seem to dominate the upper half of the house, the more hostile ones control the nether regions.

This is, after all, where each and every corpse went as it awaited the medical examiner and his crew. Negative energy was allowed to swell and gorge itself on the stale air of this basement until only those spirits bathed in darkness were left to remain in the corpses' absence. Down here, investigators, visitors, and even Todd Wolfe himself have been pushed, punched, and scratched. There was even an instance when a dark entity attacked a worker in the crawl space and sent him to the hospital with a neck injury.

EVPs that have been recorded in the basement indicate an Intelligent Haunting, with specific answers being given to specific questions asked by investigators at the time. But one doesn't always need a digital voice recorder to hear the disembodied voices of those who have passed. Down in the basement, soft, yet clear, whispers can occasionally be heard.

There seems to be no end in sight for the haunting activity at Clovis Wolfe Manor, a place that paranormal researchers call "a black hole of paranormal activity." Todd Wolfe offers haunted tours on a regular basis, but has recently revealed plans to turn Clovis Wolfe Manor into a forty-bedroom haunted hotel. Getting people to Clovis Wolfe Manor is the easy part. Getting them to stay the whole night in George or Mary's room might just be the real challenge.

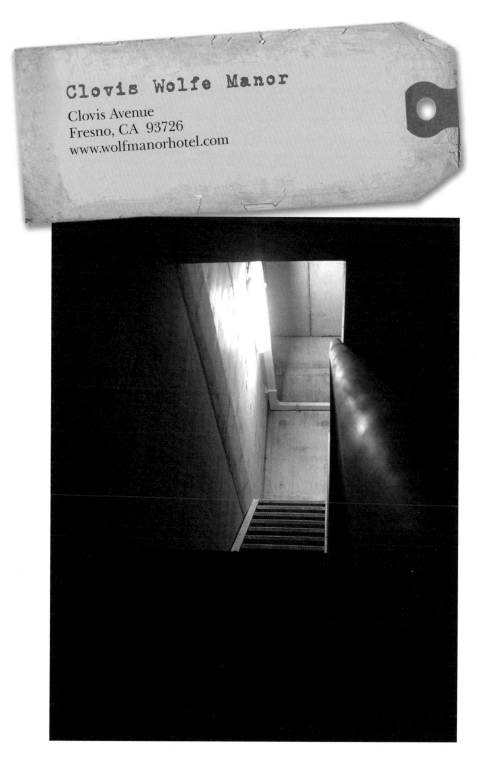

Clovis Wolfe Manor

Clovis Avenue
Fresno, CA 93726
www.wolfmanorhotel.com

PHOTO 60 - STAIRWAY

20.

BURLINGTON COUNTY PRISON
Mount Holly, New Jersey
1811-1965

"You seized that moment to plant the fatal dagger into her bosom—perpetrated the horrid deed. She lived to say 'Oh mother, mother, I screamed and you did not come, and Clough has killed me because I would not marry him!' I wish not to extract the dagger from her bosom and plant in your own. I know your blood will not atone for hers. Banish then from your mind any hope and expectation—put out at once the faintest ray of hope that may penetrate your cell and prepare to meet your God."

~Judge Hornblower to Joel Clough
July 1833

One shouldn't feel too sorry for Joel Clough. Even though he was a mere 28 years old when he faced the gallows at the Burlington County Prison, there can be no doubt that it was his own actions that put him there. And it is his own anger and rage that keeps him there, trapped forever behind those tall stone walls, an endless tormentor of the living in the quiet little town of Mount Holly, New Jersey.

Built in 1811 entirely out of brick and poured concrete, the prison was constructed to not only be fireproof, but destruction proof as well. Architect Robert Mills assured everyone involved that would-be rioters would have a dickens of time setting fire to the place or tearing it up. In essence, it was an indestructible fortress that withstood everything until its closing in 1965. Originally structured to house only forty prisoners at a time, the warden's house was built neatly next door and connected to the prison with an elaborate tunnel system. Cells were outfitted with fireplaces and that was it. No bed or lamp, no chairs or basins. Prisoners of similar dispositions shared their cells with each other, and women were segregated and tended to by the warden's wife.

This was how it was when Joel Clough arrived in 1833, sentenced to die on the gallows for murdering the daughter of his former landlord. This was, by no means, Joel's first brush with the law, nor was it the first time he had reacted out of anger. Clough was the youngest of seven children, and by Clough's own admission, was the most spoiled. His parents never told him no, and if they did, he threw massive temper tantrums until they gave in to him and awarded him what he wanted. By the time he was fourteen, he had started his life of crime by burning down the barn of an apple farmer who had caught him and his friends stealing apples. He was never punished for the crime; the fire was blamed on an errant lightning bolt that crashed during a ferocious thunderstorm.

Clough was quick to anger, always reacting first and thinking last; he would challenge his own friends if he thought they were cheating at cards, attacking them with whatever blunt or sharpened object was closest at hand. So it is hardly a mystery why, when Mary W. Hamilton twice refused his hand in marriage, Clough reacted as he did.

Mary W. Hamilton had been married to a Doctor Hamilton when she met Joel, who, at the time, was a lodger in their home. When Dr. Hamilton suddenly died (an act that gets no elaboration in Joel Clough's book), Clough set his sights on the beautiful, auburn-haired widow. It was only out of a skewed sense of social obligation that Mary paid any attention to Clough at all; she never intended, nor ever entertained, the idea of marrying Clough. She even had an 8-year-old daughter with her now-deceased husband that she wanted to shield from Clough. But Mary was his and Clough wasn't going to take a refusal.

He had asked her twice before for her hand in marriage, and twice before she had rebuked him. Clough decided that, if she refused him again, he would stab her to death with the very dagger she had given him as a gift. No one can fault Mary Hamilton for rebuking Joel; manipulative and psychotic, Joel Clough was seen for who he was by Mary. She saw the violent temper for herself and was fearful of him, afraid to spend her life and her daughter's life in servitude to a psycho.

When she refused him a third time, Clough lost it and did as he promised. He stabbed her to death in front of her sister, Elizabeth, who begged him to stop. It wasn't until Mary had taken her last breath that Clough's rage subsided and he realized what he had done. According to his autobiography, Clough felt saddened and remorseful. But his long history of violence and his hair-trigger temper make it hard to empathize with this cold-blooded murderer.

Arrested and charged with her murder, Clough was incarcerated at the Burlington County Prison, but managed to escape. When he was recaptured seven miles away, Clough was chained in the dungeon until his trial when he was found guilty and sentenced to hang. The reading of the verdict had begun at 12 noon, but the Judge wasn't able to finish until almost five that evening. Several times during the reading of the verdict, Clough interrupted Judge Hornblower, begging for clemency and mercy. Each time, he was refused. On July 26, 1833, Clough was led to the gallows behind the Burlington County Prison and hanged. His body was buried on the prison grounds, where it lies still.

But Clough's spirit roams all over Burlington County Prison, unhindered by flesh and propelled forward by his boundless anger and rage. Shortly after his death, guards and inmates alike heard moaning and the sounds of rattling chains coming from his old cell. He has claimed the prison as his own and does not take kindly to those who disrespect his so-called authority. Visitors to the prison have heard his voice near his old cell at the end of the hallway. Unfortunate women have had the terrifying experience of seeing his ghostly arms reaching out for them from between the bars of his cell door. Elsewhere in the prison, workers have seen quick, darting shadows in the dungeon and the apparition of a "legless" man floating through the air. They also claimed to see apparitions and items levitating in the cell.

During restoration of the building in 1999, workers reported strange events such as loud noises, voices, and massive drops and spikes in temperature. Items such as drills, hammers, and paintbrushes would disappear, only to appear in rooms the workers had never entered before.

In the realm of electronic voice phenomenon, several instances of "Get Out" and "No" have been recorded, in addition to the eerie murmurings of nondescript whispers and groans. Footsteps and clanking chains echo throughout the prison. Intelligent responses to investigator questions, the amount of activity that surrounds Clough's old cell, and the increase in activity around the anniversary of his hanging all point to Joel Clough's restless ghost, and he does not show any sign of relenting.

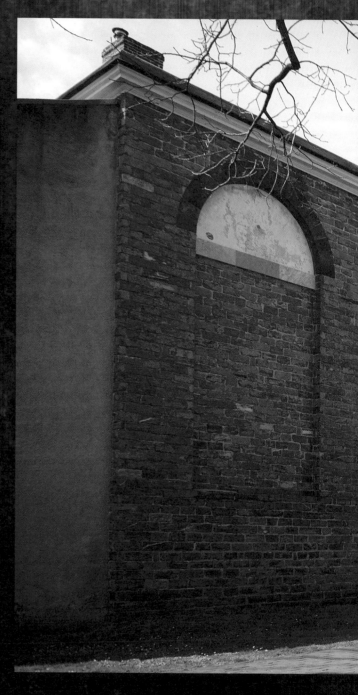

The Burlington County Prison in Mount Holly, New Jersey. *Photo courtesy of Kevin Husta, Owl's Flight Photography.*

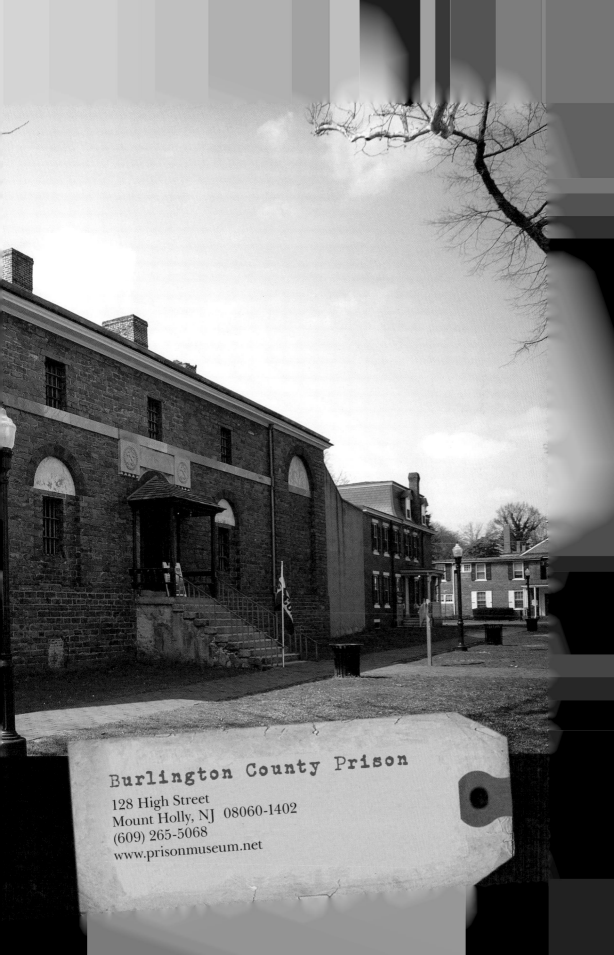

Burlington County Prison

128 High Street
Mount Holly, NJ 08060-1402
(609) 265-5068
www.prisonmuseum.net

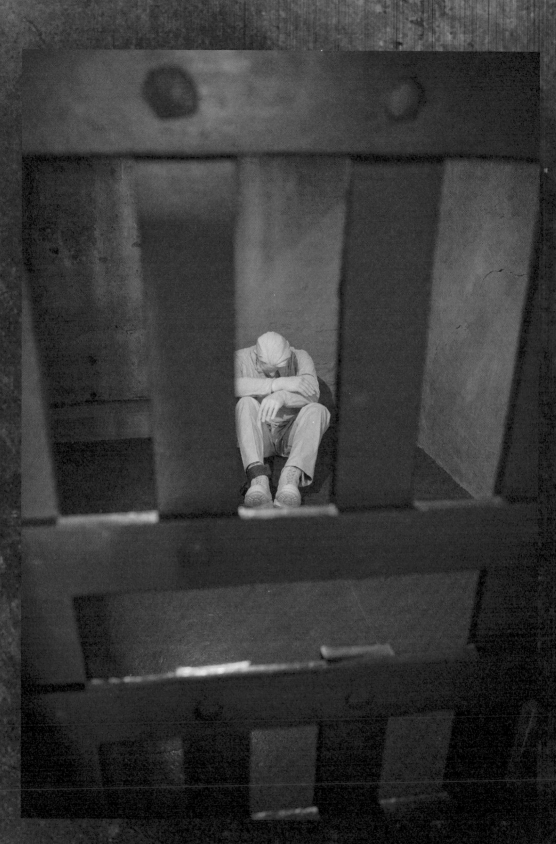

PHOTO 71 - CLOUGHS CELL DSC0077
Joel Clough was remanded to this cell and chained to the floor following his escape attempt.
Photo courtesy of Kevin H., Owl's Flight Photography.

21.

PENNHURST STATE SCHOOL
Spring City, Pennsylvania
1908-1987

"Pennhurst was a monster of a state school. There was the bumbling bureaucracy with its proverbial blindness to abuses; the aging doctors who might or might not take seriously cases such as these; the paltry attempts at school classes, sports, and recreation; the dirt, the vermin, the heartless scrimping; and, most of all, the physical and mental abuse dished out by hard-boiled and mercenary caretakers and supervisors."

~Swami Yogeshananda
Six Lighted Windows

It is, without hesitation, the shame of Pennsylvania, an institute so foul and repellent that just the mere mention of Pennhurst State School conjures up images of abuse, neglect, intolerance, and terror. For thousands of men, women, and children, Pennhurst State School was supposed to be a safe haven from the cruel tortures of the outside world. But they had no idea that what lay beyond the doors of Pennhurst State School was worse than what the world could possibly conjure.

Quite literally, the Pennhurst State School began life with a stigma attached to it already and the insensitive nature of the school was revealed when its true first name was unveiled: Eastern Pennsylvania State Institution for the Feeble-Minded and Epileptic.

In 1903, the Pennsylvania Legislature created a commission to organize and take census of those mentally and physically disabled. This commission discovered that the state's almshouses, insane asylums, and prisons contained no less than 3,773 mentally and physically disabled persons. It was enough reason to alleviate the population at said institutions and create a new institution designed specifically for the needs of the disabled. The design of the property would include two buildings: one for educational and industrial purposes, and one for non-parental custodial care and for the insane. Provisions were made for no less than 500 patients with room designated for additions should the need arise.

From 1903 to 1908, the first of the buildings was constructed on 634 acres in Spring City, Pennsylvania. Included in the first buildings were the boys and girls dining halls, kitchen and store room, three cottages for female patients, two cottages for male patients, living quarters for teachers and staff, a school, and an administration building. A massive campus, indeed, and there was more to come. By the time construction came to a close in 1930, an additional twelve buildings had been added, including a green house, power station, and a treatment plant.

In November 1908, the first patient was admitted to Pennhurst. Patients were classified into categories, whether they were merely slow or insane, epileptic or healthy. After only four years, Pennhurst was already overcrowded and they were under pressure from local lawmakers to start accepting immigrants, orphans, and criminals. But in a rare display of foresight, the superintendent at the time had this to report to the Board of Trustees.

It is without question absolutely wrong to place the feeble-minded and epileptic in the same institution. They are not the same; they are as different, one from the other, as day is from night. They are mentally, physically, and morally incompatible, and require entirely different treatment.

The mission of the institution was clarified and only people with mental disabilities were to be admitted. Luckily, the patients were spared the terror of sharing their space with the criminal and insane elements. Or so they thought.

Overcrowding quickly became an issue, as rooms designed to house three to four patients now had to be used to house up to ten patients at a time. It got so bad that beds were lined up in such a way that the patients could not get in or out in the traditional manner. To the children who lacked proper reasoning skills, they opted to soil themselves rather than attempt to navigate across ten crib-like beds to the bathrooms. In turn, the orderlies and nurses forced to clean up after them began taking out their frustrations upon the children in the forms of beatings.

Psychologists were not on duty, nor were they on-call, at night or over the weekend. When patients had a crisis, they were left to their own devices, strapped to their beds or just plain ignored until the next morning or until the weekend was over. Physical restraints became a substitute for staff because of shortages in funding or employment and there were cases of several patients who spent months in restraints, aggravating their already fragile emotional states even further. Urine and feces commonly littered the floors, as did the occasional pool of blood when a patient would hurt him or herself enough to bleed. What's more is that, while Pennhurst was supposed to be preparing patients for the working world outside, it was proven very well that the patients were *not* schooled at Pennhurst, and even began to lose the skills they had learned on the outside. Patients were allowed to beat and assault their fellow patients; the complete list of injuries sustained while Pennhurst State School was open for business would have filled a 300-page book.

Former patient Roland Johnson, in his autobiography *Lost In A Desert* says:

It sounded like vibrations: crazy people was going out of their heads, out of their wits.... It just sound like people that need to belong there. It sound to me, in my personal feeling, that people was just doing things that should not have happened. So that's what it sound like; it sounded like... fear; that something was not right. It was just scary—a frightened, scary place.

Not only did the patients learn to fear one another, but the people they were supposed to trust and put their faith in took extreme advantage of them and their fragile mental and emotional conditions. Staff members beat, neglected, berated, and even raped and sexually assaulted the patients in their care. If a patient was considered a "biter," his or her teeth would be pulled out, often without sedation. If a patient was known for being a "wanderer," then he or she would be tied or shackled to their beds or the radiators in their rooms. Nothing was off limits. For the patients at Pennhurst State School, death was a relief. The real horror came from living. Pennhurst State School had become a living Hell for thousands of innocent victims.

Finally, in 1968, television news journalist and NBC correspondent Bill Baldini aired his expose of Pennhurst State School on the local NBC10 news. Presented in five parts, "Suffer The Little Children" ripped the lid off of Pennhurst's violent and psychopathic practices. While sterilization no longer seemed a viable treatment, segregation from society was. Shipping the retarded and the mentally ill twenty-five miles out of town, away from much of a society that would shun or exploit them was as much for our benefit as it was for the children's.

"These unfortunates are being deprived of their dignity and self respect," commented Baldini in his expose. "Why? Because only a very, very few seem to care." But Baldini was quick to assert that the negligent treatment of the children was not the fault of the doctors, nurses, or orderly's working at Pennhurst; rather, it was the massive under budgeting the State of Pennsylvania had allotted to the hospital. For example, the Philadelphia Zoo had been allocated just over $7 a day for the care of each animal by the state. In comparison, Pennhurst was allowed just over $5 per child for care, feedings, and education.

"The children—who are rotting in their cages, cribs, and beds—can thank society for their dreadful plight," said Baldini. "We have forsaken them, not in the sense of what we have done to them, but by what we have failed to do on their behalf."

That mentality of stunted budgeting by the state limited aides and doctors to one for every hundred patients. The ordeals at Pennhurst were a result of a collective ignorance, beginning at a state level and trickling down to the janitors and groundskeepers.

The expose described in vivid detail all of the horrors, violence, neglect, and corruption the patients at Pennhurst had to endure on a daily basis. To the patients and their loving advocates, it was as if salvation had finally come to them. But to Pennhurst, it was only the beginning.

Still, the ordeals of the children at Pennhurst weren't always the result of conscious actions of the staff. Many kids were, in fact, treated harshly because that is how society embraced the mentally ill.

The airing of "Suffer The Little Children" immediately gave way to a flurry of inquiries, finally coming to a head in 1974 with a class-action lawsuit against Pennhurst State School. Three years later, U.S. District Judge Raymond J. Broderick found Pennhurst guilty of violating patient's constitutional rights. They were forced to close in 1987 following several more allegations of physical and sexual abuse. All 460 patients were transferred to other facilities or discharged entirely. Oddly, Pennhurst was made responsible for discussing treatment plans with each patient's family in an attempt to decide what would be best for the patient.

While it was open, the sounds of screams and torment were deafening, radiating for miles out into the Pennsylvania wilderness. When employees or visitors arrived, they were met with raucous, often bloodcurdling screams and shouts from the hundreds of children confined inside. But when Pennhurst closed, the sudden and stark silence became an eerie and haunting sound.

Since the closing, many ideas have passed in and out regarding Pennhurst's future. Some wanted the place torn down and a Veteran's Cemetery erected in its place, others have offered to use it as a place of commerce or habitation. Still, there are a great majority of people who would rather see it used as a beacon for understanding, as a memorial for those who suffered there, and as the school of higher learning it had set out to become.

Today, it stands empty, with a few of the buildings undergoing renovations, including the Administration Building, which is being retooled into a haunted attraction. Wisely, the developers have agreed to respect the wishes of the public and are relegating their haunted attraction to only the administrative wing, and not the patient rooms or dorms. Finally, the respect and dignity they begged for had come at last.

But with the renovation process came the uncovering of some truly unsettling things. Workers began to hear voices of children crying, screaming, and yelling. Doors slam everywhere and the uneasy footsteps of former patients echo throughout the long corridors. Soft thuds of ghostly heads banging against the walls, broken and disjointed voices call out for their mothers, and the infrequent, yet chilling appearance of white, vaporous apparitions near the tunnels below.

The Tunnels

Deep in the basement of the main building at Pennhurst State School lies an elaborate tunnel system connecting the main building to all of the surrounding out-buildings. The tunnel system allowed employees access to all of these buildings, as well as providing a covert exit for patients being transferred from one building to another.

It also provided access to the Morgue, which sat near the entrance of the tunnels. Of all of the 5,000 people who died here, this was their last stop before being transferred to a funeral home.

Dark and labyrinthine, the tunnels provided those predators who worked for Pennhurst a place to take their unwilling victims. Molestations, rapes, and other sexual assaults reportedly occurred in the tunnels at the hands of a patient whose spirit has apparently returned there following his death. Investigators and visitors often report the presence of a malicious, ill-tempered spirit who pushes, punches, gropes, and, in the form of EVPs, has sworn repeatedly in a deep, grisly voice.

Elsewhere in the tunnels one can hear the sound of footsteps, the crying of children, and chilling laughter from deep within. Most times, the sounds get tangled, and one isn't certain from which direction they are coming, adding to the creepiness of an already creepy place.

The Quaker Building

While Pennhurst was open, the Quaker Building was used to house the worst of the worst: children so emotionally crippled and physically violent that the patients were treated more like inmates, with restraints, quiet rooms, and solitary confinement cells. This was also one of the more bloody buildings, with murder and suicide occurring on an almost daily basis.

It has been said that more apparitions appear here than in any other building. Most of these spirits have been seen in the upper rooms, looking out the windows into the courtyards below. Witnesses have seen dark figures pulling curtains apart, their eyeless faces looking down upon stunned witnesses. Upon further inspection, it was discovered that a wire mesh covers the entire berth of the windows—curtains and all. Human hands could not have moved the curtains, and drafts of air are uncommon.

To many mediums, Pennhurst isn't merely a former institution. It is a ghost factory—a mass grave so full of spirits that one needn't walk too far inside without running into one. Atrocities against helpless children, whose treatment Pennhurst's employees blame on lack of funding, still stain the hearts of those who survived it and those who did nothing to stop it. Over the years, the negative energy has been draped over this place and hangs heavy to this day, attracting the darkness that now calls it home.

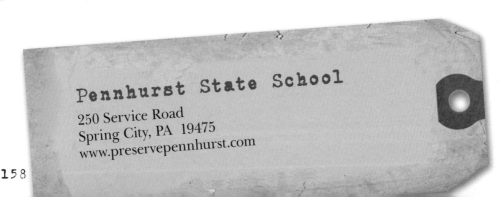

Pennhurst State School
250 Service Road
Spring City, PA 19475
www.preservepennhurst.com

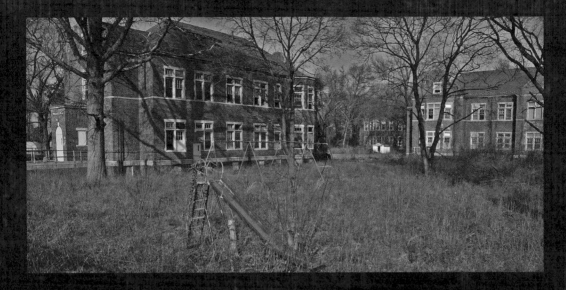

PHOTO 79 - PLAYGROUND
The abandoned playground. *Photo courtesy of Ryan Wirth.*

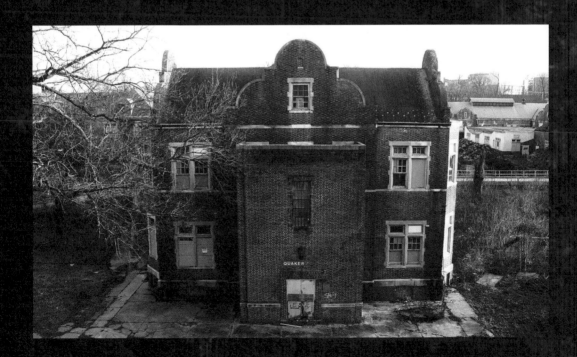

PHOTO 80 - QUAKER HALL
Quaker Hall, the most haunted building at Pennhurst State School. *Photo courtesy of Ryan Wirth.*

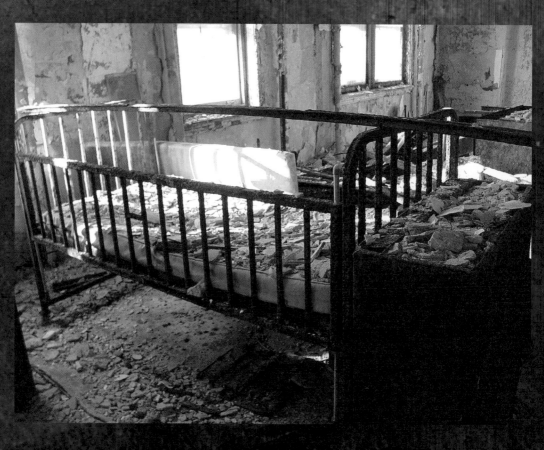

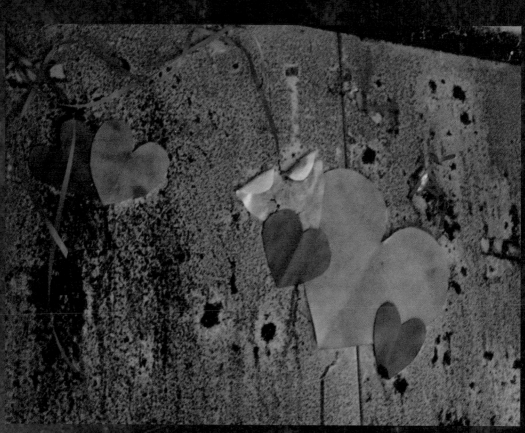

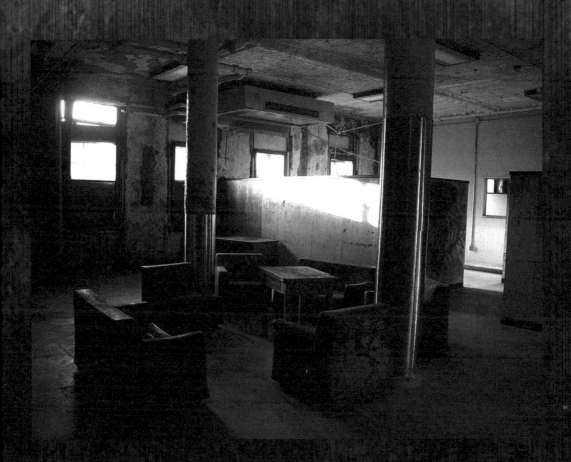

PHOTO 78 - PENNHURST DAY ROOM
This day room, while empty and quiet now, would often be filled with possibly hundreds of mentally challenged and disturbed children. *Photo courtesy of Ryan Wirth.*

PHOTO 111 - PENNHURST CRIB BY HANNAH CHERVITZ
Photo courtesy of Hannah Chervitz.

PHOTO 112 - PENNHURST HEARTS BY HANNAH CHERVITZ
Paper hearts, cut out by Pennhurst students for a Valentine's Day celebration, still cling to the rotting walls they were pasted to so long ago. *Photo courtesy of Hannah Chervitz.*

22.

FORT LEAVENWORTH MILITARY BASE AND
DISCIPLINARY BARRACKS
Leavenworth, Kansas

"Jails and prisons are designed to break human beings, to convert the population into specimens in a zoo—obedient to our keepers, but dangerous to each other."

~Angela Davis

Aside from the Federal Prison and United States Disciplinary Barracks, Fort Leavenworth has become an entire city unto itself. Were it not for the walls surrounding the fort, one might mistake it for any other old town in Kansas.

One of the oldest and most feared prisons in the United States, soldiers facing court martial prayed they didn't become incarcerated at Leavenworth, and those who did face their incarcerations there returned to civilian life with tales of brutal, gut-wrenching experiences with discipline and punishment. They also tell stories of eerie goings on: full-bodied apparitions, weird noises, and lights. Former guards and employees share stories of phantom guards in the towers and hallways, as well as the spirits of executed prisoners wandering about the graveyards.

Civilian prisoners, on the other hand, found their lives changing at Leavenworth's Federal penitentiary, a prison run by the Federal government and usually housing the nation's worst of the worst. Most were holders of a life sentence, though those who were only to serve a few years were sent to Leavenworth because they may have been disciplinary problems or known for violent outbursts.

The military portion of the prison was built in 1874, housing military prisoners and prisoners of war. Common convictions ranged from insubordination, desertion, and fraud, to murder and treasonous activity. By 1895, the Department of War transferred ownership of Leavenworth Prison to the Department of Justice, essentially creating the Nation's first Federal prison, a place for offenders convicted of crimes against the United States.

A new facility was built around 1919, beginning with the obligatory cell blocks and offices. Shortly thereafter, bakeries, shoe shops, and other textile manufacturing buildings were constructed and made a part of the new Federal prison. Prisoners were transferred out of the original prison, and it was returned to the Department of War, where it became the United States Disciplinary Barracks (USDB) at Leavenworth.

So now, with a civilian Federal Prison at Leavenworth and the original military prison four miles down the road, the history of crime in America was about to get a little bit more colorful. Over the years, the Federal prison at Leavenworth housed such notable inmates as Robert Stroud, the Birdman of Alcatraz; gangsters "Machine Gun" Kelley and "Bugs" Moran, who died a month into his incarceration of lung cancer; American Indian activist and poet Leonard Peltier; and, more recently, disgraced NFL player Michael Vick. Even James Earl Ray, assassin of

Martin Luther King, Jr., did time at Leavenworth for forgery before his more famous crime was even committed.

Like most prisons in the world, the murders of guards and inmates alike, as well as the high-strung tensions of serving in the military, creates an environment ripe for both Intelligent and Residual Hauntings. One of the more interesting stories came from a former guard at the military prison, whose identity he wisely kept to himself. Twelve towers lined the perimeter of the prison, with only Tower #8 remaining unmanned. Yet, while on patrol in his own tower, this officer who was stationed at the prison while in the army, received numerous phone calls from Tower #8. It was reported that shadowy figures could be seen inside the tower, even though no one had ever stepped foot inside. He even received calls from other guards in other towers who reported that someone was trying to get into Tower #8, knocking and banging on the door. But when he would look out the window, the guard would see nothing there. Rumor has it that a soldier killed himself in Tower #8 and that his ghost still roams the perimeter. Records regarding suicides amongst American soldiers are held close to the chest, so discovering the identity of this poor man who felt he had no other recourse is difficult indeed. But if you believe the legends, he walks the halls still, always on patrol, still serving, still vigilant, but obviously very lonely.

Inside the walls of Leavenworth, there is a whole slew of buildings, all serving different purposes. Building #65 had once been used as the hospital, but now serves as a health clinic, dentist office, and barber shop, as well as a housing unit for minimum-security prisoners. It is believed that fourteen German prisoners of war had been executed in the unused elevator shaft of Building #65. Soldiers patrolling the building at night have reported hearing bloodcurdling screams coming from the bottom of the elevator shaft.

Elsewhere in the hospital, workers and inmates alike have reported seeing a ghostly duo of patients, one pushing the other in a wheelchair down the hallway outside of the infirmary. Patients in the hospital have even been woken out of sleep by a mysterious patient in a wheelchair who disappears almost as soon as he makes himself known.

A Mothers Eternal Search

At the National Cemetery on the grounds of Leavenworth, reports have been flying regarding the phantom of a woman named Catherine Sutter, draped in a black shawl, wandering amongst the tombstones—a true "Woman In Black" tale.

The story goes that, in 1880, Catherine, her husband, Hiram, and their two children, Ethan and Mary, stopped at the recently opened Fort Leavenworth on their way to the Oregon territory. It is said that their two children disappeared one day while collecting firewood for the family and believed that they were swept into the nearby river and drowned. A search yielded no results and by the time winter arrived, the search for the children had to be given up and Ethan and Mary were presumed dead. The Sutters stayed on through the winter, hoping that the children would find their way back. Catherine would often be seen walking through the snow and woods, calling out to her children.

The hours of wintry searching took their toll on Catherine, who contracted pneumonia and died during that winter at Leavenworth. Devastated, Hiram Sutter returned home to Indiana, where he soon received word that his children were, indeed, alive. They had been swept into the river, as hypothesized, but were rescued by a band of Fox Indians on a hunting party. They had been taken back to the Indian camp and given food and shelter through the winter before being returned to Fort Leavenworth in the more mild and less harrowing spring. Tragically, the ghost of Catherine Sutter still wanders the National Cemetery, still looking for her children, still lost and trapped in this world, still separated from her beloved family after all these years. She has been seen carrying a lantern, and at other times, her ethereal voice is heard on the wind, echoing throughout the darkness of the cemetery.

The Officer's Quarters

On McClellan Avenue sits the prestigious Officer's Quarters, a place for visiting and attending officers to relax, unwind, and maybe tell a ghost story or two—possibly about the ghost that haunts the very building in which they are staying. Legend has it that the face of a man appeared along the back brick face of the fireplace, watching and staring at the living officers, lingering there until the fire had all but nearly died out. His mustachioed face still provokes memories from those who heard the tale and passed it down, for this man has made more than just the random one-off appearance at the back of the fireplace.

He's also been seen in the upstairs bathroom, readying a razor and soap for shaving. Some even believe he's been heard, as phantom footsteps loudly pummel the wood floors and heavy doors slam shut on their own at all hours of the day and night. Who is he? No one knows. Plenty of officers have lived and died at Leavenworth; it's almost impossible to tell. Whoever he is, he surely enjoys the accommodations.

Father Fred

The St. Ignatius Chapel sits on the corner of McClellan and Pope Avenue on Fort Leavenworth's post, but the original chapel burned to the ground in 1875, situated on land that is now a private residence. A tragic accident, the fire claimed the life of the young priest, Father Fred, who worked and lived at the chapel.

Although the chapel was a total loss, what material could be salvaged was salvaged and used to build the home that sits on the property to this day, including a large number of scorched bricks. It is said that Father Fred still ministers on the property, appearing as an apparition clad in his priest robes and collar as he walks through the house. His heavy footsteps can be heard on the stairs and in the dining area, day or night. Perhaps most intriguing is a Polaroid photo taken in 1973 that revealed the blurred image of a man dressed in priestly robes.

Sumner Place

At 16 and 18 Sumner Place, a rarity has occurred. In this sprawling duplex on the Fort Leavenworth campus resides a "Spirit in Black" whose quiet demeanor and complacent disposition is a welcome change to stories of the vengeful-angry-hostile type of phantom. Dressed in black, this spectral woman has been seen cleaning in the duplex and attempting to help with the daily chores.

Supposedly, she was a nanny and maid who served the homeowners of the neighborhood at one time or another. Her calm appearance makes her a draw for children; many different children have told their parents about the nice lady in black who would tell them stories or sing them to sleep. A most helpful spirit, this mysterious woman's only mission, it seems, is to continue to serve the families who choose her house to live in.

The Rookery

Just across the way on Sumner Place is the oldest house in Kansas, a simple little home known as The Rookery. Built in 1832 with timbers dating back to the Revolutionary War, The Rookery has seen its share of famous guests, including Nathan Boone, son of Daniel Boone, and General Douglas MacArthur, who was a mere captain when he stayed there.

Quite simply, The Rookery *is* the most haunted house in the entire state of Kansas. The vast number of recorded experiences with a wide variety of different spirits is well known and the statistics are enough to validate the claim of "Most Haunted in Kansas." The Rookery has been inhabited ever since its construction and has seen a lot of lives begin and come to an end.

One of the more prolific spirits is said to be that of an older woman with long hair who runs at people with her long fingernails, hands poised in a clawing-type attack. Rumor has it that she may have been the victim of a domestic violence situation, though there is no proof to this claim, only hearsay on the part of my sources. Without a doubt, the ghost exists. How she got to be that way is the question no one can answer.

Other experiences tell of an elderly woman who prefers to stand motionless in the corner of the front room; the only sound coming from her is the chattering of her teeth. Could this be the spirit of a woman who may have died of hypothermia, possibly due to the brutal winters of Kansas?

A third and fourth apparition reported are that of a young girl and an old man. The young girl has been seen, and heard, throwing a temper tantrum throughout the whole building. The old man, on the other hand, tends to rouse other men from sleep. One of the more defining characteristics of this shade is the bushy hair on his head; it's the one thing people who are wakened by him seem to remember.

The Sheridan House

Located on nearby 611 Scott Avenue, The Sheridan House was built by General Philip H. Sheridan as a home for he and his common-law wife, Harriet Lindsay. Nothing is really known of Harriet, except to say that she may have been an Indian woman and that the two were not legally married in the eyes of the government.

Because Sheridan had many dealings with the Indian tribes of the Plains and put down many rebellions, Harriet may have been a gift to General Sheridan, a gift that he wanted to send back but couldn't. In any case, it has been reported that Sheridan wasn't exactly kind and loving to his young wife. He left her in 1869, traveling to Chicago after being promoted to Lieutenant General, while she toiled on her death bed with typhus. What is interesting is that Harriet Lindsay did not die. She languished in abandonment until her death in 1933 at the age of 94. It is said now that her ghost haunts her old homestead, seeking revenge upon men in general, not just her former husband. Men have woken with scratches on their bodies, felt burning stares from the darkness, and heard indecipherable whispers that sounded more like rabid scoldings than the more genial spectral voices one normally hears.

Harriet Lindsay is a woman scorned, and Hell hath no fury that can match her feelings of betrayal and loss. For the men who venture in Sheridan's House, its best to give her a little space.

Fort Leavenworth Disciplinary Barracks is a fully functioning and operational federal penitentiary. They do not give tours and I wouldn't push my luck trying to visit, if I were you.

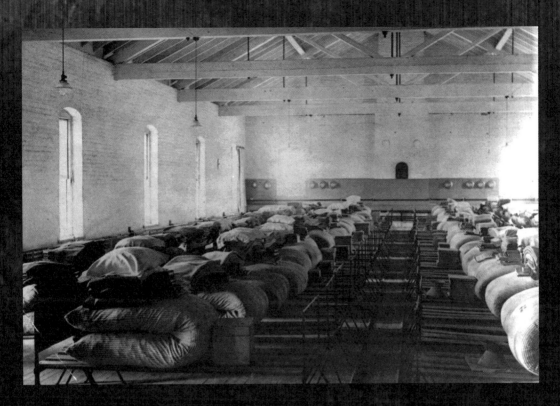

PHOTO 7 - LEAVENWORTH PRISON DORM 1910
The dormitory of Leavenworth Disciplinary Barracks, 1910

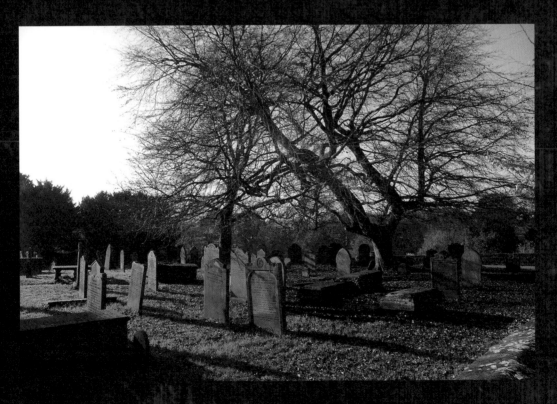

PHOTO 4 - BURIAL GROUND

23.
THE ASYLUMS AND HOSPITALS OF INDIANA

"Now I know what a ghost is. Unfinished business, that's what."

~Salman Rushdie

Madison State Hospital
Madison, Indiana

In the extreme south of Indiana, near the banks of the Ohio River, sits an asylum the locals used to refer to as "Cragmont" (because it is situated on Cragmont Avenue). The Madison State Hospital was established in 1910 in an effort to alleviate overcrowding at the state's other institutions, as well as to more properly serve the mentally damaged from the southern portion of the state.

Consisting of twenty cottages and an administration building, the Madison State Hospital began life as the Southeastern Indiana Hospital for the Insane with its first patients newly arrived from the overcrowded Central State Insane Asylum in Indianapolis. Transported by train, the patients were guarded by security armed with shotguns filled with rock salt. What they found at Madison's new hospital was a breathtaking view of the Ohio River, lush woods and a serene atmosphere that exuded calm and peace. To the architects and administration, the view from the windows and porches of the hospital was just as important for mental recovery as the new drugs and therapies being touted in mental health in those days.

Over the years, like many institutions, many people saw their ends come at Madison State Hospital. Suicides and murders were as common there as they were at other places, and like those other places, ghost stories began to abound.

One particular story revolves around a disturbed old man who walked off the grounds and tried to make an escape via the nearby highway. He was killed when he jumped in front of a car in an attempt to flag it down. Today, when driving down that same stretch of road, some people have claimed to see the old man try to flag them down for a ride. But when they slow the car to a gradual halt, the old man vanishes from sight, leaving nothing behind but a deep chill down the spines of everyone in the car.

Another variation of this tale involves seeing the old man in the woods surrounding the hospital. While out on a moonlit walk through the woods, a young man and his girlfriend encountered an old man dressed in pajamas and a robe. His hair was disheveled and his eyes conveyed that of a damaged, almost wounded soul within. To the young couple, he looked out of place in the chilly woods. Before they could say anything to him, he simply turned and started to walk away from them, slowly vanishing in the night.

Needless to say, the young couple opted to take a different route the next time they felt like taking a walk in the woods late at night.

The Indiana Veterans' Home West Lafayette, Indiana

Along the heavily wooded path known as Soldier's Home Road in West Lafayette, Indiana, lies one of the more majestic, crowning achievements for the continued health and welfare of Indiana's revered veterans: The Indiana Veterans' Home.

The campus itself sits on more than 250 acres of beautiful, wooded hillsides that seems almost too removed from the bustle of the Purdue University campus, not five miles away. A massive, Arlington-like cemetery houses the resting bodies of soldiers who have fought in every major American war since the Civil War. The ghosts of brave soldiers and nurses alike are said to still wander this placid, serene place of healing.

Built in 1896 in an effort to better care for the returning Civil War soldiers and their families, the Indiana Veterans' Home quickly became known as a haven for America's soldiers who returned home from conflicts at home and abroad. Still in operation today, the Veterans' Home has seen its share of tragedy, hope, and redemption, and that is evident in the souls who choose to remain at this place, a place where they found peace and healing.

According to former coworkers, the Pyle Building, a residence hall for the veterans, is said to be the most haunted building on the campus. Numerous employees, both past and present, have reported the eerie running of the building's elevator. The doors will open, and no one will be inside. Other times, it is said that the specter of a nurse exits the elevator, the appearance of which always seems to coincide with a death somewhere in the building of one of the residents.

Both residents and employees have had experiences in the Pyle Building that still chills their blood to this day. Many have reported being touched and hearing faint whispers in their ears, all perpetrated by unseen forces gliding through the hospital corridors.

A former nurse's assistant posted her own story about the hauntings in the Pyle Building on StrangeUSA.com, saying that she was visited by an unseen force while cleaning up a deceased resident. The assistant felt a hand on her shoulder and her name being whispered into her ear. But when she turned to see who it was, no one was there.

Also of note is the Commandant's House, a large, fully restored house on the property that once served as the residence for the Commandant in charge of The Veterans' Home during the earliest days of operation in the late 1880s. Today, it serves as a fairly prestigious Bed and Breakfast. But one gets more than a good night's sleep and a tasty meal in the morning.

Those who have stayed at the Commandant's House have reported the sounds of ghostly footsteps roaming the hallways in the dead of night, and a well-uniformed officer of the Civil War has been spotted walking around the property at all hours of the day and night.

Being a resident of the Lafayette area for my entire life, I myself have heard stories of lonely soldiers, garbed in both battle fatigues and crisply pressed uniforms, wandering about the rows and rows of white cross headstones, as if searching for someone they once knew. They move slowly and silently through the graveyard for several moments until, finally, they disappear into thin air.

It is my belief that there is nothing malevolent or sad about the Indiana Veterans' Home. Some came into the Home because they were haunted by what the war had done to them. With great care and hope, they found the serenity they had been searching for all along. It is a quiet, peaceful place of healing that retains its souls not because they are trapped, but because they want the peace to last forever. I can't say I blame them.

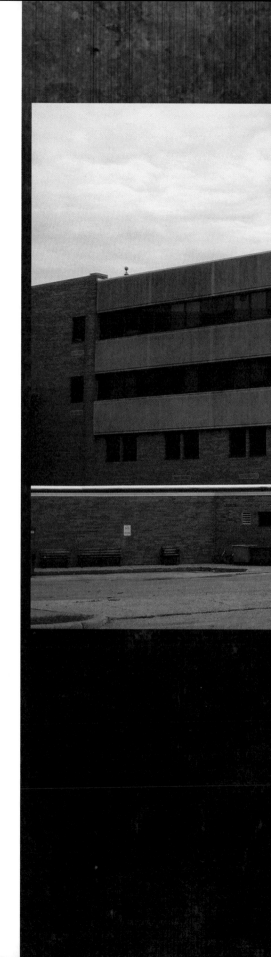

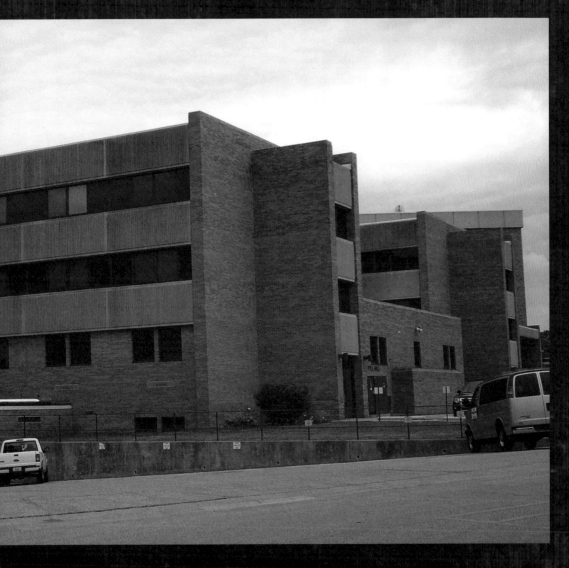

PHOTO 102 PYLE BUILDING
The Pyle Building of The Indiana Veterans Home in West Lafayette, Indiana. *Photo courtesy of the author.*

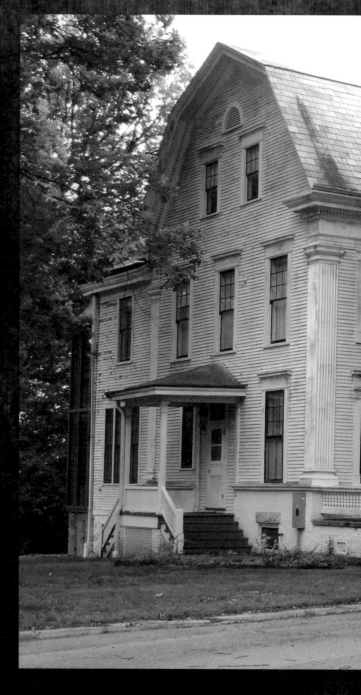

PHOTO 103 - COMMANDANTS HOUSE
The Commandants House. *Photo courtesy of the author.*

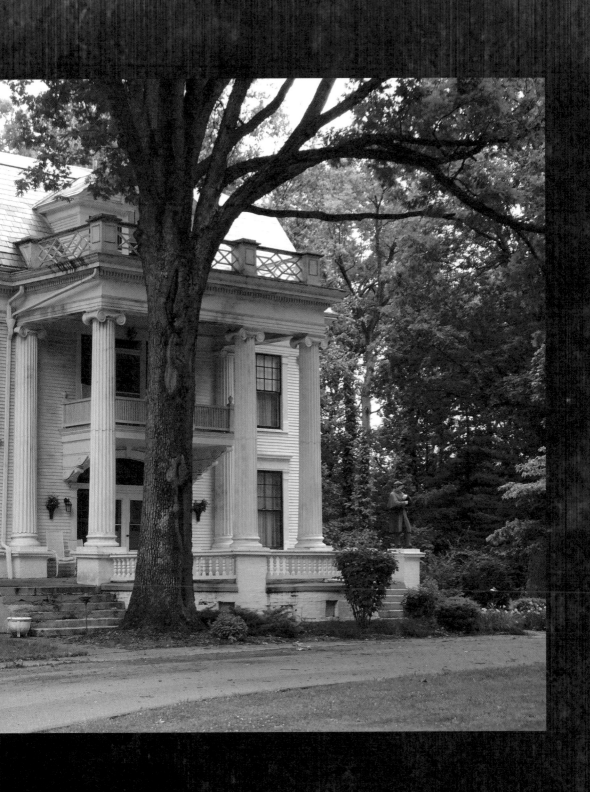

24.

OLD CHANGI HOSPITAL
Republic of Singapore
1930-1997

"Don't matter if you believe in them or not. If they're there, they're there."
~Joan Lowery Nixon

Most Asians believe that there are not separate worlds for spirits and humans; rather, it is one big world that is shared by both, a place where the dead roam as freely as the living. Ghosts and spirits are as common as sunshine and there is always a very real fear that a ghost or spirit will cling to you and never let go. People place religious symbols in their homes, not as an affirmation of faith, but as a means of protection from evil.

Places like the Old Changi Hospital in Singapore are reflections of that very old philosophy. Located on the Netherveron Road in the village of Changi, the old hospital was built in 1930 to service the people of the village. But during the invasion of China, during the infancy of World War II, the forces of Japan seized control in a bloody siege and took control of the Changi buildings, making the hospital their headquarters.

From there, the legends of torture, death, and horrific executions began to take root. Rumors of the brutal treatment of Chinese prisoners of war cast fear into the hearts of the villagers. But the brutality of the Japanese would be paid back in full when World War II came to an end. The Japanese soldiers were hunted down and taken to their own deaths in the places where their fellow villagers were cut down.

The military barracks that were left behind were converted into hospital rooms for the public portion of the hospital. In 1994, the Changi Hospital officially moved out of the village and relocated. Seated on a hillside, it was far too rough on patients and employees to continue to fight going up the steep flights of stairs. The buildings that were left behind became havens for ghosts and demons who, according to villagers, roamed about freely, unencumbered by pesky humans. The ghosts of the past reclaiming their graveyards and tombs...*this* is how the villagers see it and this is why they are wary of treading upon those grounds. It was also during this transition that the rumors of hauntings began to circulate.

Villagers told tales of ghostly Japanese soldiers stalking the Changi streets after dark, wearing the all too familiar Imperial Guard uniforms seen during World War II. It was a scary thing, but one that people merely accepted as an inevitability of the actions that took place during the war. To the superstitious people of Singapore, being haunted is the price you pay for dishonorable lives.

One of the more interesting sightings that villagers have claimed is the sighting of the dreaded Pontianak, a so-called Malaysian vampire. The Pontianak usually appear as pale women with long dark hair. They emerge dressed in white and take on a comely appearance so that men might be ensnared. Some claim that the Pontianak was invented by Malaysian wives to discourage their men from engaging in random sexual encounters with strange women. Once a man is engaged, the Pontianak rip open their prey and devour their organs.

This myth of a black-haired female demon is a common folktale amongst the people of Asia. The Chinese believe a black-haired maiden named the Yuan Gui stalks the night searching for revenge upon those who killed her. The Yurei of Japan have a very similar appearance to the Malaysian Pontianak and the Yuan Gui of China: long flowing black hair covering much of the face except the eyes, which are terrifying and full of despair. The Yurei and Pontianak myths are thousands of years old and are still frightening people to this day; their legends inspired the vengeful ghosts of JU-ON (*The Grudge*) and RINGU (*The Ring*.)

In the case of the Changi Hospital, the Pontianak have reportedly been seen wandering about the grounds, appearing and disappearing at will, and it is said that those who encounter the Pontianak are never seen again.

As I stated before, the ghosts of Japanese soldiers have been seen wandering about the grounds, but natives to the area have also seen the specters of Chinese mercenaries and soldiers, caught, tortured, and ultimately executed by their Japanese captors. Still others report seeing the ghosts of Caucasians, possibly the spirits of British soldiers who failed to repel the Japanese in the battle over the Malaysian peninsula during World War II. Brave visitors to the Old Changi Hospital have also reported seeing the ghost of a baby crawling across the floors and the spirit of an old Chinese woman with long white hair in a dilapidated wheelchair.

According to a former patient who goes only by the name Ah-Toh, he had seen—and smelled— firsthand these eerie goings on even while the hospital was open for business.

During my two weeks stay, I saw occasional shadows moving about on the ceilings of the corridor when it's empty, and heard some coughing near me, even though I'm the only patient in the ward, during days and nights. There was once I woke up to a strong flower perfume on a particularly cold night. Tried everything: increase the speed of ceiling fan, rub tiger balm near the nose. The perfume disappeared when a nurse came in during a routine check.

Ah-Toh's story isn't unique. Numerous patients, trespassers, and ghost hunters alike have reported the same things. But what about the security guards who work at the government-owned building? Well, they're another story altogether. A guard identified only as Mr. Tan was interviewed by Singapore Paranormal Investigators and was asked about the Changi Hospital being haunted.

I even slept here, never [have] see[n] any ghost before. I also never heard of anybody [who] went missing here or anybody [who] jumped down from the building as what the rumors wrongly said.

The ghostly activity of the Old Changi Hospital even extends out to the beaches surrounding the hospital's mountainside location. It was here, on these placid beaches, that tens of thousands of Chinese citizens and sympathizers were executed, beheaded by Japanese soldiers because they refused to swear allegiance to the empire of Japan.

Today, it has been said that spectral bodies will wash up on the bloody shores of Changi Beach, heads grotesquely missing. Others claim that the heads themselves can be seen flying through the air, as if lopped off in a quick, sudden movement.

To the citizens of Changi Village and the Singapore government, demolishing the buildings and rezoning the land is not an option. Destroying the buildings would either anger the spirits or send them out into the world. Nobody wants either of those alternatives. For now, the Changi Hospital buildings will stay, yet remain empty, save for the hundreds of souls who call it home and the thousands of villagers intent on keeping their distance from this bloody and haunted place.

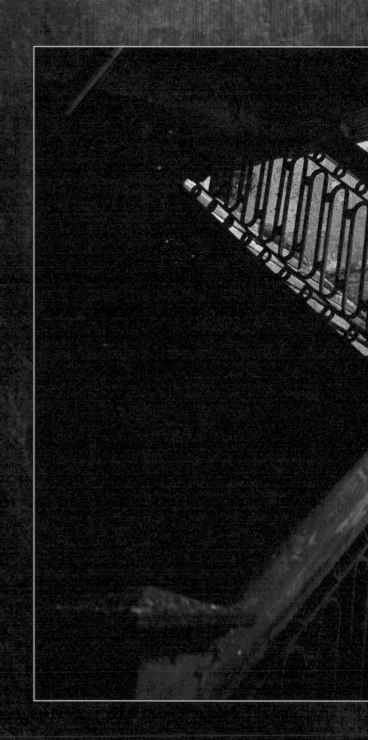

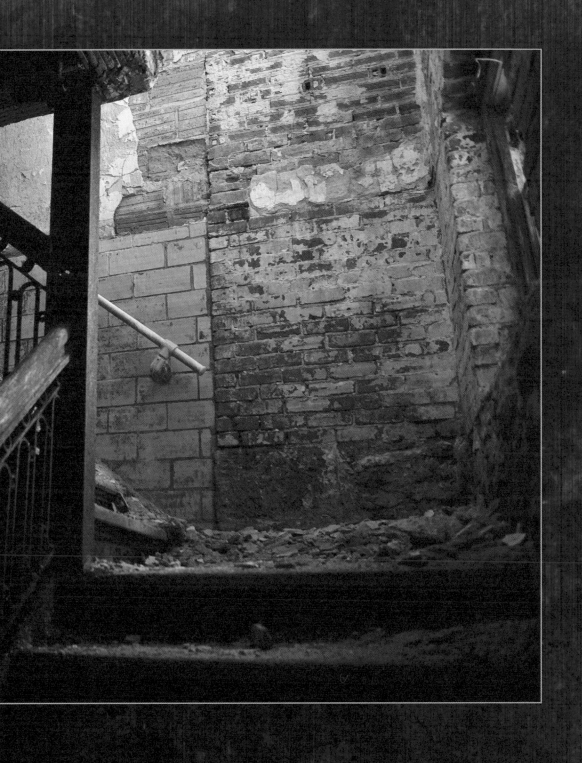

25.

POVEGLIA ISLAND
Venice, Italy
421 AD-1963

"Sickness shows us what we are."

~Latin Proverb

Locals refuse to go near the Island in the daylight, let alone during the nighttime hours. Fishermen avoid it like the plague. Most everyone who knows of it believes it to be cursed. Parapsychologists and investigators alike have deemed it one of the darkest places on Earth.

Welcome to Poveglia Island.

Located at the fringes of Venice, Italy, surrounded by the deep blue waters of the Mediterranean Sea, lies what may possibly be the closest thing to Hell on Earth for the living of the world. To some Italians, Poveglia Island is an evil, dark place that brims with the tormented souls of centuries past. To others, it is a place good only for storage, and the only ghosts that walk there are the ones in the imaginations of others. While some Italians discount the paranormal activity and other Italians play it up, there is little doubt amongst ghost hunters, mediums, and even the skeptic tourist that Poveglia Island is perhaps the most haunted place in the world.

Poveglia Island was first found in historical documents around 421 A.D. when the peoples of Padua and Este fled to escape the hordes of barbarian warriors bent on conquering the tiny countries. By the 9th century, Poveglia had become incredibly populated by the descendants of the Paduans. As its importance in the region became more and more important, it was decided that it should be governed by a Podestà, the Italian version of a governor who answered only to the Emperor of Rome. But with Poveglia's importance in Italy came the risks of others wishing to control the island.

Barbarian hordes still made their presence known, as did the nearby armies of Genoa. Despite their victories over the invaders, the people of Poveglia moved off of the island and an octagonal fortress was erected, fittingly called "The Octagon."

Even after the building of the fortress, the island remained uninhabited. For an island so many wanted to control, no one wanted to step foot upon its shores anymore. The Camaldolese Monks were offered the island as a monastery, but they refused it. Even the descendants of the original inhabitants refused to return. One can only wonder, with that proverbial chill racing up and down your spine, what happened to make so many refuse to return? It could be that it was a magnet for battles and bloodshed, or was it the presence of the new angry spirits of the slain invaders?

In 1777, something happened that sealed Poveglia's reputation as a place of death and suffering. The island had come under the authority of Italy's Public Health Office, who used Poveglia as a checkpoint for goods and people coming into Venice by ship, a place much like Ellis Island had been for the United States. It was during this period that several members of a sailing party revealed themselves to be sick with the Plague. As a result, the island was transformed into a confinement station for the sick, or a Lazzaretto. It continued in this tradition until 1814, when

Napoleon Bonaparte shut it down so that he could use the island to store his huge cache of weapons and artillery.

Sometime during the early 20th century, it was again used as a quarantine station, but closed a short time later. By 1922, the existing buildings on Poveglia were converted into Viennese retirement homes. These lasted until 1968 when they were closed, citing waning use. Combined with a severe lack of agricultural prospects, the island was left alone once more.

Those are the facts. But here are the stories, those tales that are just as true, but not as flattering as the Italian government wants them to be.

During the 14th, 15th, and 16th centuries, as the Bubonic Plague was crisscrossing the continents of Europe, Poveglia Island became a storage area for the staggering number of dead and dying who suffered and perished because of the Plague. The ferry boats ran in almost continuous shifts, as workers stacked bodies like corded wood into gigantic trenches known *affectionately* as "Plague Pits." Thousands upon thousands of victims were forced from their homes in Venice and tossed upon the shores of Poveglia never to return.

Over the three centuries that the Plague was active, it is estimated that close to 200,000 died of the disease and faced their death alone on Poveglia Island. Today, thick layers of gray ash, lining the upper crusts of Poveglia's surface serve as a reminder of the fiery Plague Pits of days gone by. The sheer number of corpses was so great that Venetian fishermen still find human bones amongst the fish in their nets, dredged up from the bottom of the lagoon.

In 1922, after the outbreaks of Plague had passed and World War I had come to a close, some of the buildings were converted into a mental institution and a retirement community, a story that grants Poveglia Island its inclusion into this book of haunted prisons and asylums. In 1963, all functions on Poveglia Island were stopped, the buildings abandoned, and the remaining patients and residents were shipped off elsewhere. In time, the Italian government took control of Poveglia and has restricted its access to most people. According to many, its main use today is said to be as a place of storage. Not that you could find anyone outside of the paranormal community willing to go there, and it is certain that Poveglia isn't good for anything but harboring the dead and their remains anyway.

The Bell Tower

Near the retirement home on Poveglia Island is a soaring Bell Tower that, when it served as a monastery, would call the monks to worship. But during its day as a retirement home, it quickly became known as the starting point to one of the most chilling ghost stories to ever come from Poveglia Island.

It all began in the 1920s when the resident doctor, one Dr. Damyan Nikolovich, began to notice marked changes in his elderly patients. Many of them began to experience the same delusions, hallucinations, and deliriums. Dr. Nikolovich classified those patients as suffering from what is now called Phasmophobia, an intense fear of ghosts, and he compounded that diagnosis by classifying them as suffering from Phantasmagoria, which is the delusion of seeing ghosts. The patients relayed story after story of seeing these dark, angry spirits, hearing threatening whispers in their ears, and smelling the scent of burning hair and skin. Certainly, to a doctor of reason, they all must have been suffering some sort of group hallucination brought on by legends of Poveglia's sinister past.

But somewhere along the line, the good doctor snapped. The experimental treatments he practiced on his patients in order to cure them became torturous, painful, and some say deadly. It is widely accepted that Dr. Nikolovich went mad, driven to insanity perhaps by the same dark energies and ghosts that haunted his patients. Experimental surgeries and treatments that bordered on absolute butchery masqueraded as therapy. His mad experiments continued until, one day, he calmly went to the Bell Tower of the hospital, climbed the 150-foot ladder to the top and abruptly fell, or jumped, to his death. Some stories say that his enraged patients dragged him up to the top of the Bell Tower and tossed him over the side, but climbing the tower ladder is difficult for one man, let alone one being dragged kicking and screaming by multiple men.

Still other stories say that it was a priest, not a doctor, who jumped from the Bell Tower window, a permanent solution to a temporary loss of faith.

Whichever story you choose to believe, it is certain that someone walks the floors of the old hospital still, surrounded by the thousands of spirits who look to him for guidance, be it spiritual or medicinal. Those who have been fortunate enough to have encountered the residents of the Bell Tower and hospital recall a sinister Italian voice whispering ominously into their ears before intense headaches and nausea sets in. Objects have been thrown or tossed at people, loud bangs have broken the silence of the decrepit hospital, and unexplained spikes, as well as drops, in temperature are all said to be signs of the spirits' presence in the ruins of the Bell Tower.

The Burning Grounds
and The Plague Fields

The ground at the north end of the island drank gallons of blood and swallowed thousands of bodies, leaving powdery ash and bone fragments behind. It was here, along the North Coast of Poveglia that the "Plague Pits" lay, massive trenches dug out of the Earth and filled to the brim with the corpses of Plague victims. Fires consumed the bodies of men, women, and even children in an unending blaze that was kept well fed.

The grounds near the eastern side of Poveglia, however, held the Plague Fields, a large open field where sufferers of the Plague spent much of their days and nights, waiting for the end to come. The only cure for these unfortunates was death, and death dealt with the dying harshly. Guards and doctors policed the fields, assessing the victims regularly. If a patient seemed to be close enough to death, they were taken north to the Burning Grounds and tossed onto the flaming pyres. Their screams of terror and horrendous pain could be heard near the shores of Venice as they burned to death. For three centuries, this practice remained in place until, finally, the Bubonic Plague was considered extinct.

Imagine the horror of knowing how painful your death will be from the Plague. Imagine the awfulness of knowing that, once you reach Poveglia, you will never see your home or family ever again. Imagine the terror of being hurried to the north end of the island, where flames wait to consume your living flesh and smoke and fire become your breath and blood. The spirits who live on Poveglia Island suffered that and remained on Earth as wrathful ghosts, resentful of the living who are able to come to Poveglia and leave with their lives.

White, mist-like apparitions have been seen crossing the Plague Fields in the dead of night, unimpeded by the tall grasses growing up around them. The distant voices of the dead have been heard mingling with the wind as it whips through the lagoon. Loud footsteps on wooden bridges have been heard very clearly. EVPs of men, women, and children have been captured by the scant number of paranormal investigators lucky enough to explore the island and escape with their evidence.

To the north at the Burning Grounds, expect to see much of the same thing, but the residual smell of burning hair and flesh has been known to waft into the unwilling nostrils of those fortunate enough to survive the trek through the dense woods. Chilling screams are heard wailing through the night air, cutting through you to the bone and festering inside your soul.

Shadows and faint balls of amber light dart about the landscape, staying away from direct sight, remaining off to the sides in one's periphery. Here on Poveglia Island, you don't *think* you see something. You *know* you saw something...and something saw *you*.

A Dark Spirit Stalks the Hospital

According to most psychic mediums who have either visited Poveglia or channeled it, the single most overpowering aspects of the island are the hundreds of thousands of voices crying out in pain and terror. In addition to the hundreds of spirits residing on Poveglia, there is also the possibility of a very pronounced dark entity, possibly called up from the depths by the nonstop bloodshed and terror experienced over the years.

This demonic entity wanders about the island, unfettered by boundaries or spiritual restraints. It feeds off despair and fear and will pursue those who defy spiritual protection. Of course, there is no proof that demons or demonic entities actually exist, but would you want to take that risk, especially in a place as evil and rancorous as Poveglia? The demonic entity will feed off death and pain, and possession may not be out of the question.

Great spiritual care should be taken when visiting Poveglia or any other haunted place. You may walk in with one soul, but leave with two.

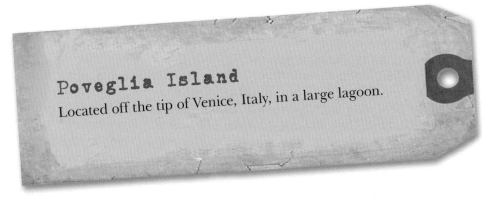

Poveglia Island
Located off the tip of Venice, Italy, in a large lagoon.

Owned by the government of Italy, tourism is strictly forbidden and the public is not welcome on the island in any capacity. Unless you're a buff ghost hunter with an American TV show and American money. (In other words, no trespassing.)

26.

COVENANTERS PRISON AND GREYFRIARS CEMETERY
Edinburgh, Scotland
Est. 1561

"Repentance is a magistrate that exacts the strictest duty and humility."
~Lord Clarendon, Edward Hyde

After the famed Edinburgh Vaults, Covenanters Prison and the Greyfriars Cemetery is widely considered to be the most haunted and terrifying place in all of Scotland. On an ancient island rife with dark history and steeped in ghostly folktales and legends, the haunting of Covenanters Prison indeed tops the list in terms of experiences rampant with sheer terror.

It is perhaps the most tragic and terrifying place to visit in Edinburgh, Scotland, with its tale of devoutly religious monks persecuted by Roman Catholic and Episcopalian armies and the crazed magistrate who set out to put an end to them and their insolence in the face of the King of Scotland. Such passages of events are the breeding grounds for dark legends and eerie tales of ghostly experiences that have spanned generations.

The Covenanters were a sect of Presbyterian monks who defied Charles the First's decree that the Monarchy ruled by Divine Right, a theory that dictates that God chose Charles the First and his successor, Charles II, personally to lead the country of Scotland's Roman Catholic Church. It was a move mirrored by the monarchs of England and Spain. But in 1638, a large group of Presbyterians banded together in defiance of this decree, arguing that only Jesus Christ can be the spiritual head of the church, not a monarch.

Prepared by Alexander Henderson and Archibald Johnston and revised numerous times over by other Covenanters, it became the official decree of defiance known as the National Covenant. Signed by thousands of Covenanter loyalists in Greyfriars Church in 1638, with thousands more names added after that, the National Covenant was copied and distributed freely amongst the people of Scotland and England. The movement of the Covenanters' had begun.

The Roman Catholic Church of Scotland enacted a period of severe religious repression against the Covenanters. Ministers and priests who fostered sympathies for the Covenanters were forced from their churches by authorities. Those who continued to preach the Covenanter philosophy faced the possibility of execution by the state, and citizens who did not attend church services were heavily fined, classified as rebels against the church, and tortured. They would be asked to take various pledges, declaring their loyalty not only to the king, but to also accept him as the Divine head of the church. Those refusing to take the oath would be summarily executed by roaming bands of mercenaries who scoured districts of Scotland in search of rebels.

These harassments became more frequent and definitively more cruel with the ascension of Charles II to the throne of Scotland in 1660. More and more Scots began to band with the Covenanters and, as a result, more battles and encounters with Scottish Government troops happened.

Finally, in 1679, at the Battle Of Bothwell Bridge, the Covenanters' army was defeated and over 1,200 prisoners were brought to Edinburgh. Roughly a quarter of them were returned to Greyfriars and imprisoned in their own churchyard; chains held the gates closed and guards ensured no one would escape before they could stand trial for treason against Charles II.

They were kept under guard for five months during the winter with minimal rations of bread and water, and little shelter from the freezing cold weather. Some Covenanters were granted their freedom after swearing an oath to Charles II. A few took up the offer, but most did not. Instead, they remained imprisoned, loyal to their beliefs. Many Covenanters died in their prison and were buried in the neighboring churchyard of Greyfriars in a spot usually reserved for criminals.

Then, after five months, those who survived their incarceration faced a far more formidable foe than the winter weather and meager rations. Sir George Mackenzie, a minister responsible for enforcing Charles II's policy opposing the Covenanters, arrived at the prison. He was a King's College educated aristocrat who led quite a distinguished life as a Lord Advocate for the throne of Scotland. He alone was the driving force behind the establishing of Scotland's Lord Advocate Library in Edinburgh. But in 1680, he became known for something else entirely.

Mackenzie immediately distinguished himself amongst the Covenanters as a ruthless man who could very rarely ever be swayed by the lamentations of his prisoners. Over the course of only a few months, he relentlessly executed each surviving Covenanter prisoner by hanging. According to historians, Mackenzie reveled in his job, taking great delight in the pain and suffering of those rebellious, yet pious, Covenanters. Because of his near jubilance at executing close to 800 prisoners, Sir George Mackenzie quickly became known by another, more chilling moniker: "Bloody" George Mackenzie.

And so, following the defeat of the Covenanters, the Covenanters' Prison was shut down and returned to its first duty as a churchyard butting up to Greyfriars Cemetery. Ironically, following Bloody Mackenzie's death in 1691, he was buried in Greyfriars Cemetery, placed just feet away from the place where he'd ordered the hangings of 800 prisoners of religious war. He was laid to rest in a black mausoleum with heavy wooden doors, sealing his body away from the world.

So begins the tales of the haunting of Covenanters Prison and Greyfriars Cemetery.

The Legacy of the Covenanters

"Those with heart conditions and women who are pregnant aren't allowed into the prison itself."

Those words, eerie in tone as well as in function, are spoken by tour guides outside of Covenanters Prison to the mob of curious sightseers. It is an agreeable term. Such horrific attacks and terrifying encounters have happened inside the stone walls of Covenanters Prison—so terrifying in fact that it is a small miracle that it is even opened at all. But for those lucky few who pass the initial test of the tour guides, they get to enter and enjoy a frightening world of the paranormal most do not get a chance to see. Those others who dared to tread onto the grounds of the Covenanters Prison after dark can expect to see the dark shadows of the former Covenanters, fleeting shades that dart about the old crumbling shelters that once served as their prison.

Many tourists and visitors to the Covenanters Prison report icy blasts of cold air blowing over them, as well as fits of nausea and shortness of breath. Ghost hunters have recorded EVPs of men speaking in thick Gaelic accents and ectoplasm-like orbs have been filmed and photographed amongst the ruins.

This is splendid evidence and may be the bread and butter of a ghost hunter's life, but it pales in comparison to the horrors lying in wait in the Black Mausoleum.

The Mackenzie Poltergeist

The general feel of Greyfriars Cemetery and the Covenanters Prison used to be one of peace and gentleness, even after the bloody history perpetuated by Sir George Mackenzie. Covenanters Prison and Greyfriars remained genuinely quiet until one day in 1998. It sounds like the premise to a wonderfully scary movie, but the reality of what happened—and what continues to happen—chills the blood and freezes the soul.

Many Scottish tour guides, tourists, scholars, and parapsychologists insist that during the renovation of Mackenzie's tomb, an ancient evil was released upon the hallowed grounds of Greyfriars, one that continues to haunt the cemetery thirteen years after the terror began.

One story of how the haunting began starts with an innocent schoolboy who hid out in the Black Mausoleum in order to evade a headmaster at George Heriot's School. Supposedly, the boy lost his mind and went insane after being confronted by the ghost of Bloody (or "Bluidy," as the Scottish papers referred to him) George Mackenzie. Still another story concerns a homeless man who broke into the mausoleum searching for a place to sleep on a chilly night. As he snuggled into the coffin inside, the rotting wood suddenly gave way and the homeless man was covered in the dust of a 400-year-old corpse.

Still another tale, and one probably closer to the actual truth, goes that the haunting began when renovations commenced on the black mausoleum that was Bloody Mackenzie's resting place since his death in 1691.

Whatever the origin of this fantastic tale may be, there is no denying that something dark and disturbing dwells within the Black Mausoleum. Tourists who have visited the prison and churchyard cemetery sometimes report scratches, nausea, and the massive wallop of invisible hands. They have blacked out, been chased by pitch-black shadows, been overwhelmed by feelings of dread and horror—and it happens more often than one can imagine.

Jan-Andrew Henderson, a guide who runs ghost tours of Edinburgh, used to pause at the Black Mausoleum with his tours and became overwhelmed at the number of people who walked away with broken fingers, deep red scratches, a feeling of blacking out, and the general nausea attached to demonic infestations.

"I've even had phone calls from two people who say their partner has now been committed," Henderson adds, "and blame it on the ghost."

Since 1999, there have been 350 documented attacks and 170 people have been reported as collapsing or "blacking out." Noses have been bloodied, they have been pushed, pulled, and beaten. Dead animals have been found strewn across the property. Fires have started mysteriously on their own. Even the surrounding homes have reported poltergeist activity, all beginning in 1998, and all linked to the spirit that dwells inside the Black Mausoleum, final resting place of Bloody George Mackenzie. Henderson's own home burned to the ground one day, an act the former skeptic now blames on the Mackenzie Poltergeist.

In 2003, something happened that should have angered the spirit to no end. Its wrath should have been unquenchable, but, strangely, no retaliation from the unseen entity has been reported. According to the *Edinburgh News*, two teenage boys broke into the Black Mausoleum and stole the skull of George Mackenzie, an act that surely would have enraged the spirit.

> No doubt the ghost will be angry. The legend of the poltergeist is that it appeared three years ago when there was some damage to the graveyard and someone broke into his tomb. God knows what will happen now.

The skull was recovered and returned to the tomb, and so far, the only thing that has happened is that the Scottish government has sealed the mausoleum once more and refuses to allow anyone inside the tomb—even tourists.

Maybe that is what the spirit wanted from the very beginning. Perhaps now it is satisfied.

Greyfriars Bobby

As we prepare to leave Covenanters Prison and Greyfriars Cemetery behind, I leave you now with a tale of hopefulness and friendship beyond the grave.

This story revolves around Greyfriars Cemetery's 2nd most popular citizen, a Skye Terrier named Bobby.

In 1856, John "Jock" Gray and Bobby were inseparable. Jock was a constable for the Edinburgh police and Bobby was a stray pup he'd picked up on his beat. For two years, Bobby never left his master's side, loyal and trusting almost to a fault. But when Jock Gray fell ill from tuberculosis and died, Bobby was heartbroken. On the day Jock was buried, Bobby visited his old master at the cemetery and promptly lay down at the foot of Jock's grave.

For thirteen years, Bobby lay at his master's feet, protecting and looking after his greatest friend. Bobby was an international phenomenon, appearing in books and periodicals, even enduring photo shoots with local celebrities. When his own death found him, Bobby was granted special permission to be buried in Greyfriars Cemetery. A statue of him was erected very soon after, commemorating this most loyal of dogs. It wasn't until some time later that visitors to Greyfriars began to report seeing glimpses of Bobby near Jock Gray's plot and hearing the small bark of a terrier in the night.

In 1981, Bobby received his own headstone from the Dog Aid Society which marked his once unmarked grave. An inscription reads as follows:

Greyfriars Bobby
Died 14 January 1872
Aged 16 years
Let his loyalty and devotion be a lesson to us all.

And yes, Bobby still makes an occasional, ghostly appearance at the grave of his most beloved friend.

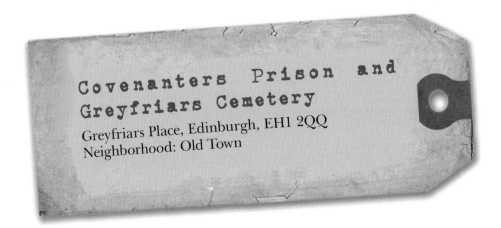

Covenanters Prison and Greyfriars Cemetery
Greyfriars Place, Edinburgh, EH1 2QQ
Neighborhood: Old Town

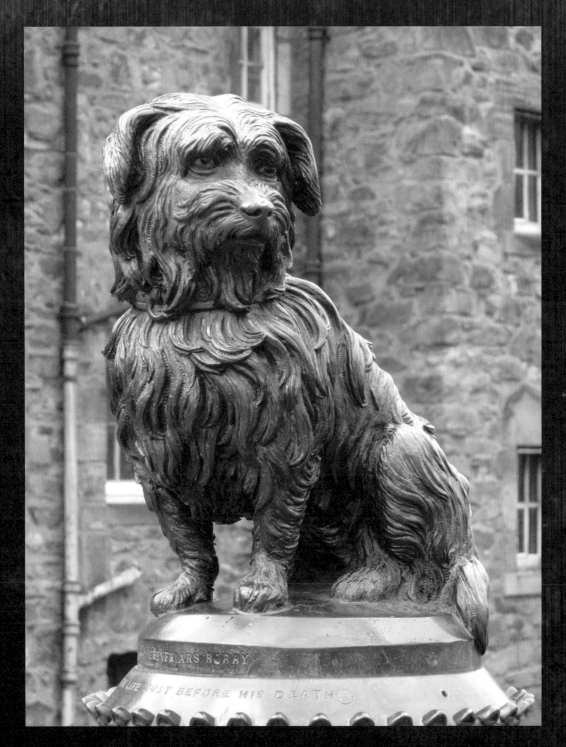

PHOTO 83 - GREYFRIARS BOBBY BY BRETT FLICK
Greyfriar's Bobby, the cutest specter in the world. *Photo courtesy of Brett Flick.*

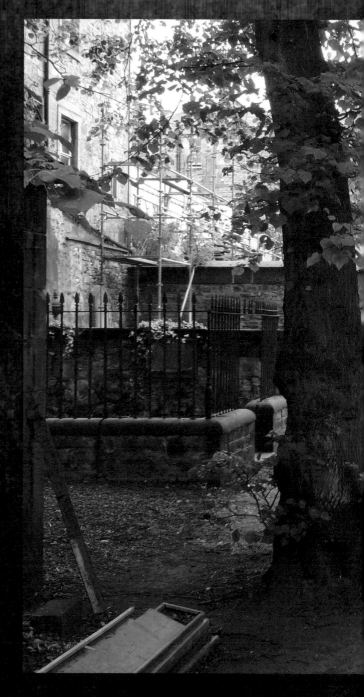

PHOTO 35 - COVENANTERS PRISON ENTRANCE

Looking in through the front gate of Covenanter's Prison and Greyfriar's Kirkyard. *Photo courtesy of Brett Flick.*

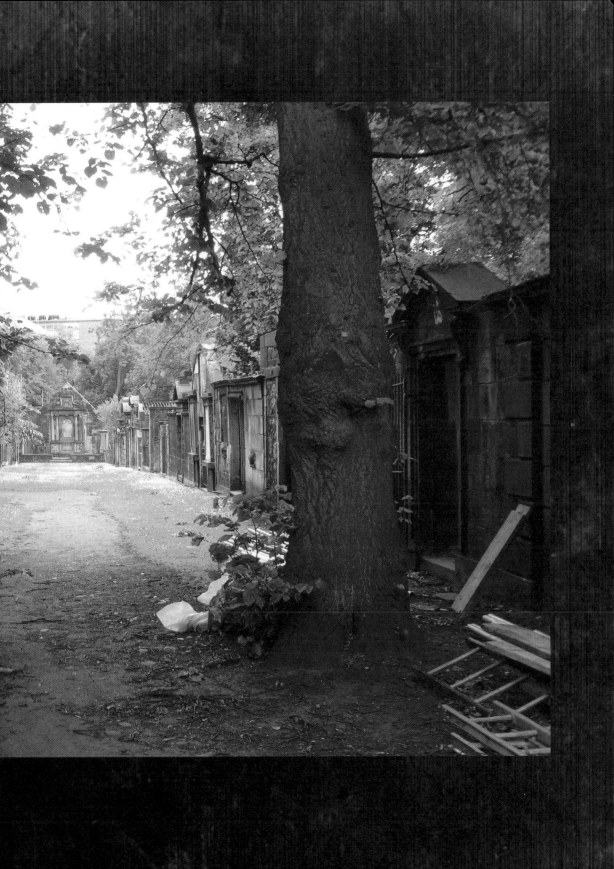

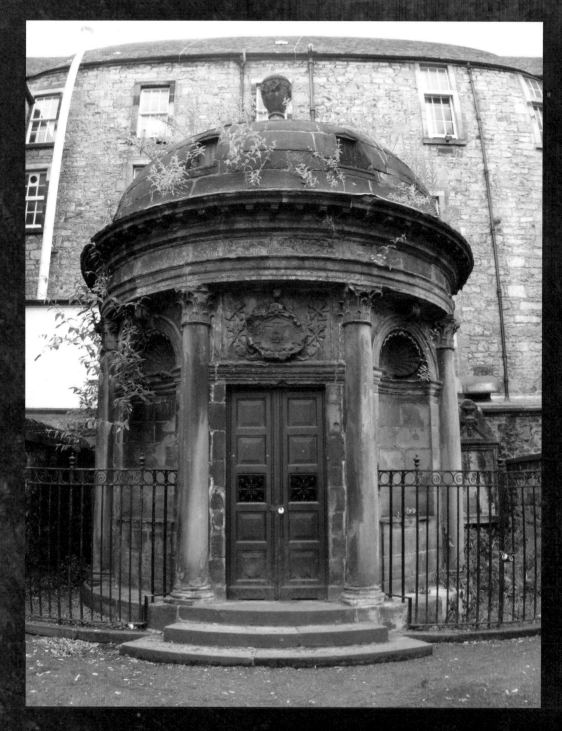

The Black Tomb of Sir George "Bloody" Mackenzie. *Photo courtesy of Brett Flick.*

27.

ABU GHRAIB PRISON
Abu Ghraib District, Iraq
Est. 1970

"The most painful thing for the inmates there were the cries of the people being tortured. One day, they brought sheets to cover the cell in order for no one to see anything. They began torturing one of them and we could hear what was happening. We listened as his soul cracked. The sound of his voice really twisted our minds and made our hearts stop."

~Anonymous Iraqi prisoner
The Ghosts of Abu Ghraib (2007)

Its name means "Place of the Ravens" in Arabic. Its horrors resonate within the United States' conscience. Images of torture and the abuse of Iraqi prisoners of war at Saddam Hussein's old Abu Ghraib prison by United States military sent shock waves through an already jaded American public and helped to further turn the tide against the war in Iraq that began in 2001 and has yet to see an end. But what the men and women of the U.S. military did pales in comparison to what was committed inside "Saddam's Torture Central" while the former dictator was enjoying the apex of his power. Few realize that before Iraq was toppled, Abu Ghraib served as the background for thousands of deaths of innocent Iraqi civilians and politicians, deaths that would ultimately lead to Hussein's execution for war crimes. In the wake of those deaths, Abu Ghraib would become home to the spirits of Iraq's tormented, tortured, and forgotten.

The prison at Abu Ghraib was originally called the Baghdad Central Confinement Facility when it officially opened in March of 1970. It was initially built to accommodate only 4,200 prisoners, but those limits would soon be tested to the point of International attention. It spans an impressive 280 acres, sports numerous guard towers, and five separate cell blocks to hold five different categories of inmates: long term, short term, foreigners, capital criminals, and those who have committed religious crimes, namely breaches in the laws of Islam. Each cell block contained eight-foot-square cells, cafeterias or "mess halls," a prayer room, and an exercise yard. Ideally, it was very much like many of the Federal prisons located in the States, and when it opened, Abu Ghraib held fast to the strict standards of the International prison system. It lacked panache, but served its grim purpose well.

But then Saddam Hussein of the dictatorial Ba'athist Party rose to power and forcibly removed the Iraqi government, placing himself in charge in 1979. Almost immediately, Abu Ghraib became the most overcrowded prison in the world. Estimates place the total number of inmates at Abu Ghraib during its peak at nearly 10,000 inmates, though those estimates seem a bit conservative. There were reports that upwards of 40 men sharing a single cell at one time. But the overcrowding was about to become the least of their worries.

The people of Iraq began to see in Abu Ghraib a new form of terror as Saddam outfitted the prison with brutal, violent guards who beat and tortured the inmates relentlessly. The prison quickly became a symbol of fear and darkness, a concrete Boogeyman. Men who were serving time for stealing bread or coveting his neighbor's wife (a serious breach in Islamic law) mingled side by side with murderers, rapists, and terrorists, especially those terrorists belonging to groups whose ideology opposed Saddam's.

Filled with his enemies, detractors, and Shi'ite loyalists, the new dictator of Iraq was also free to dispose of those who had so vehemently and vociferously opposed him. In 1984, Hussein took into custody, then ordered the mass executions of thousands of people in his widely feared "Death House," where hangings and gas chambers took the lives of over 4,000 of Saddam Hussein's people. Saddam was so proud of his Death House that he even brought his two young sons, Uday and Qusay into the prison, instructing them in the art of torture as a negotiations tactic. Uday would eventually grow up to become a certified psychopath, killing indiscriminately whenever he wanted, seemingly unstoppable until Allied troops shot him to death in a fire fight near Mosul, Iraq in 2003.

Between the years of 1984 and 2001, it is believed that Saddam had secretly executed over 500 men, most of them Shi'ite Muslims. There has also been speculation that Saddam used a great number of men as experiments in secret biological and chemical warfare tests. By the end of 2001, it was reported that Abu Ghraib housed well over 15,000 prisoners and the number grows exponentially each year. When American and Coalition forces toppled Iraq and deposed Saddam of his power, Iraqi civilians, militants, and former Abu Ghraib convicts converged on the prison, defacing Saddam's image and stole whatever they could. When mass graves were discovered near the property, it was finally understood just how vile and brutal Saddam Hussein really was. The graves contained over 4,000 bodies, victims of Saddam's Death House. Now, with Abu Ghraib in American and Coalition custody, it began to serve a newer purpose: that of a military stockade for insurgents and prisoners of war.

And then, the unthinkable happened. Pictures surfaced in the summer of 2004 of American soldiers terrorizing, torturing, and abusing Iraqi prisoners being held at Abu Ghraib for being a part of an insurgency that targeted American troops. Disgusting and horrific, the pictures showed smiling American soldiers posing with often naked and bloodied prisoners. Is it possible that the madness of Abu Ghraib grabbed hold of these soldiers? Or perhaps the madness of war turned them into the very thing they were fighting? Certainly, the parallels are eerie enough to question whether a demonic entity was at work, turning once dignified soldiers into brutal shades of their former selves. In my own opinion, the ghosts of Abu Ghraib were infecting the souls of those American soldiers, forcing them to repeat the behaviors of the Iraqi guards who perpetrated the same brand of torture upon their prisoners just a decade before.

It was during this time that the first trickles of a ghostly element made their way back to the States, with soldiers stationed at Abu Ghraib reporting that they oftentimes felt as though they were being watched, not by one set of eyes, but by a hundred sets of eyes. Soldiers would investigate scurrying shadow figures in the long corridors, only to find nothing.

The prison had quieted some and it was now calm enough to notice just how haunted it truly is. While most of the prison's hallways and cells seem to be draped with a melancholy that is as thick as wool, it is in Saddam's Death House that much of the paranormal activity takes place. While inside, one can feel and absorb the empty feelings of desperation, horror, and misery. Pictures taken inside the Death House reveal bright balls of light that materialize only on the photograph and not in real life. These "orbs" are believed by many to be the spiritual light of the ghost itself. Mist-like fog has also been photographed in the Death House, again, visible only on the picture itself. While the nooses have been removed, there is still a sense of dread and a thickness in the air near the scaffolding of the gallows.

Inside the small Death House cells, some American troops have reported to their families that they could hear disembodied whispers, voices speaking in Arabic. While only whispers, the soldiers were certain that they emanated from inside the cells as they stepped into them. Perhaps the most chilling story of Abu Ghraib's paranormal activity revolves around the elusive specter of a former prisoner who was beheaded.

The race or nationality seems to be a mystery, but the occasional appearance of a dark, mist-like figure is definitely not. It appears as a standard human-type form, but with one exception. It resembles a human figure that is missing its head. According to anonymous soldiers, this figure has been seen walking outside the prison wall near the Death House. Its appearance is so rare that many in the military believe it to be a folktale or urban legend. Perhaps it is. One could believe that. Until it shows itself again.

But the horrors of the ghosts of Abu Ghraib aren't confined solely to the prison itself. In the surrounding homes and villages, just outside the gate of Abu Ghraib, residents tell tales of ghosts and curses that have literally come knocking on their doors late at night. The mostly Sunni Arab residents of Abu Ghraib (the town) say that ghosts of Abu Ghraib (the prison) knock on their doors late at night, that the spirits make messes in the kitchens and bathrooms, that a death curse has risen up out of Abu Ghraib and now walks freely in the night, looking to eradicate purity.

Superstitious housewives in the neighborhood would tell tales of the Iraqi spirits who knock on doors and frighten their children in their dreams. Some choose to ignore it by avoiding sight of the prison; others recite from the Q'ran and pray, which they claim helps to dispel the ghostly visitations.

Superstitious or not, the facts are that school enrollment is down, over 600 acres of farmland has been left unsown for years, and as many as seventy percent of the surrounding homes have been abandoned by their owners. If it wasn't one before, the town of Abu Ghraib is now working on becoming a true Iraqi ghost town.

Abu Ghraib has now officially been returned to the new Iraqi government, who have pledged to help clean up Abu Ghraib's tarnished image at the hands of the American military. But the ghosts of Iraq's past will not rest in peace. They only wait for others to join them.

28.

THE TOWER OF LONDON
London, England
Est. 1066

What other dungeon is so dark as one's own heart!
What jailer so inexorable as one's self?"

~Nathanial Hawthorne

It rivals Alcatraz in terms of being the most well known of any prison anywhere in the world and it certainly is the oldest on our list. Its long, dark history is rife with bloodshed, deceit, betrayal, tragedy, and drama, the likes of which no one has ever known before or since. But its reputation as history's bloodiest fortress is largely undeserved because since its inception in the 11th century, the Tower of London has only hosted just over 112 executions. Its notoriety as a torture chamber, however, is unparalleled. The skill and precision with which the Tower guards practiced their art of confession seizing cruelty served as a template for thousands of monarchs, kings, and dictators all over the world.

When it was finally finished in 1078, by William the Conqueror, it was originally designed to be a palace for the Royal Family of Britain. During the 12th, 13th, and 14th centuries, expansions to the Tower were overseen by Kings Richard the Lionheart, Henry III, and Edward the First, though much of the original Tower of London has remained largely the same throughout the centuries. Looking at the layout of the Tower today, one can see several different buildings surrounded by two defensive walls and a moat. It was essentially a luxurious home for Royals, visiting dignitaries and their families, as well as religious figures loyal to the Crown. The Tower served as an armory, a treasury, and as home to the famed Crown Jewels of the United Kingdom; it was for the most part the forerunner to the as-yet-to-be-built Buckingham Palace.

It wasn't until the age of the Tudors that the use of the Tower of London began to change, favoring the uses of the dungeons and prison cells. The keepers of the torture chambers were always busy, meting out agony to the King's enemies, forcing out confessions before the prisoners were ultimately executed.

Such a case involved Guy (or Guido) Fawkes, a British soldier loyal to the Roman Catholic Church. In an odd twist of fate, Fawkes had become part of a plot to rend the British Parliament to ashes in an attempt to overthrow the Protestant influence over London. He was ultimately caught along with his other thirteen conspirators and gruesomely tortured nearly to death until he finally confessed all to his jailer. As a result, he was sentenced to be executed by hanging and by being drawn and quartered. But he became a National hero when he leapt to his death from the hangman's scaffold and plunged to the ground, snapping his own neck in the process and sparing himself the agony of dismemberment. To the people of London, he was a man who refused to allow someone else to control his destiny. Even though he wasn't the ringleader of the so-called "Gunpowder Plot," the impact of his life and death is still discernible today and his name is the most easily recognizable of the original thirteen conspirators.

Another fairly famous icon of British history that spent time in the Tower of London was Sir Walter Raleigh, a poet, historian, and explorer who was serving a sentence for a plot against King James in 1603. Despite the fact that he had a death sentence on his head, Raleigh was allowed to live with his family in the Tower and was even allowed to leave on expeditions to Venezuela, where he successfully attacked a Spanish outpost. Upon his return to England, the ambassador to Spain successfully demanded that King James reinstate Raleigh's death sentence. On October 29, 1618, Raleigh was beheaded for his initial crime against King James, his last words being, "Strike, man! Strike!"

For the most part, the Tower of London received very little maintenance over the centuries and its age was truly beginning to show by the time the 18th century began. Periodic repairs were made, but for much of the more deserving parts of the fortress it was too little too late. It wasn't until the mid-19th century that renovations on the Tower of London finally returned the former palace back into the marvel that it was.

But by then, not even renovations could erase the bloody history and the chilling stories that had now become part of the world's collective conscience. Tales of deceitful kings, treacherous royal wannabes, and the sad murders and executions of Royal England's innocent youth all added to the mysterious aura of the stone beast known as the Tower of London.

King Henry VI

May 21.

Remember that date, for the ghost of Henry VI does—540 years after his murder in the Wakefield Tower.

The only son of legendary King Henry V and Queen Catherine of France, Henry VI was never known as the most charismatic or most powerful leader the kingdom of Britain had ever known. But he was one of the brightest, having founded both Eton College and Kings College. His marriage to Margaret of Anjou resulted in her usurping the throne from him because of Henry's constant battles with insanity. His oldest son, Edward, was said to be the perfect successor to his father's reign, a prince much more suited for the throne than the weak Henry VI. His younger sons, 12-year-old Edward V and 9-year-old Richard, were too young, but should anything happen to their older brother, Edward V would ascend the throne. (Their tale is told later in this text.)

Detractors and conspirators had devised a plan to assassinate Henry VI, but they could never act upon it unless Edward was dead as well. He was imprisoned in the Tower and others ruled in his name. But when Edward was suddenly killed at the Battle of Tewkesberry, the conspirators and assassins saw their chance. Henry VI was stabbed to death in the Tower, and it has always been speculated that it was his nephew, Richard of Gloucester, who murdered the insane king in order to quicken his own rise to royalty and become King Richard III.

Now, many lifetimes later, it is said that the ghost of Henry VI still walks the corridors of his last home on Earth, manifesting only once: at the stroke of midnight on the anniversary of his death, Henry VI's ghost appears in the room in which he was murdered. By the last stroke of midnight, Henry VI is said to dissipate into the air for another year.

The Bad Death
of Margaret Pole

Margaret Pole, the Countess of Salisbury, was once an attendant for Henry VIII's wife, Catherine of Aragon, and was herself of noble blood. After her mistress' annulment from King Henry VIII was invoked, she maintained her loyalty to the King and stayed on, practicing her duties with the new Queen, Anne.

But her favor ran out when her exiled son, Reginald, a Cardinal with the Roman Catholic Church, wrote a book called *Pro Ecclesiasticae Unitatis Defensione*, a book that denounced the English King's policies. It also pulled no punches about his true thoughts concerning the King's marriage to Anne Boelyn. Because Reginald was out of Henry's reach in the country of Italy, Henry did the next best thing: he began to round up and imprison Reginald's family members, including his brother and cousin. Soon after, they were executed.

To her credit, Margaret did her best to denounce her son's book, pledging her loyalty to Henry, and even writing a letter to him condemning his actions, punctuating her pointed critique with: "I wish I'd never given birth to such a traitor."

Many of Reginald's family were arrested and executed, but Margaret, remarkably, seemed to come out untouched from the scandal. However, Henry's fear that Margaret could become the focus of a rebellion against the throne landed Margaret, now 65, in the Tower prison. She was stripped of her titles and lands, and spent an agonizing two years in the Tower. He refused to execute her, as he thought she may die of old age soon enough.

But in 1541, Henry's fears about a rebellion instigated by Margaret came true. Although she denied inciting such a rebellion of the people, Henry ordered her to be executed anyway. What happened next has been debated since the awful event took place.

One story tells of a defiant Margaret, refusing to lay her head on the chopping block, forcing the headsman to hack and slash at her with his axe as she ran across the Tower Green, screaming in terror and agony as she was brutally hacked to pieces.

The other, and possibly truer, story goes that Margaret lay her head upon the chopping block, but the chaos was caused by an inexperienced headsman rather than a defiant Countess. It is said that the headsman hacked and chopped at her head, neck, and shoulders until she was dead.

In either case, it is certain that the bad death of Margaret Pole, Countess of Salisbury, was gruesome, agonizing, and horrific for not only Margaret, but for those in attendance viewing the grim spectacle. What also is certain are the widespread stories of Margaret's return to the Tower Green as a ghost. It is said that her specter wails as she runs throughout the Green, presumably being chased by her amateur executioner, as her chilling screams pierce the thickest of London's fogs and chill even the most hardened Londoner's blood.

The Ghosts of Lady Jane and Lord Dudley

The great-grand niece of Henry VIII, Lady Jane Grey, was merely a child of 13 when she was chosen by King Edward VI, Jane's first cousin, to succeed him upon the throne of England. As he lay dying, Edward spoke publicly and put into writing his intentions for Jane to succeed him. Himself only a child of 15, his decision was met with shock and contempt for the new teenage Queen, especially since the natural line of progression would have meant that Edward's half sister, Mary, should have succeeded him. Edward's decision mystified some, and angered many.

Together with her husband, Lord Guilford Dudley, also a teenager, the two awkwardly set out to do the best job they could. They were keenly aware that older Royals coveted their position and must have known that the unorthodox decision made by Edward VI would come under incredible scrutiny.

Within hours of Edward's death, Jane was crowned the new Queen of England and she named her husband the Duke of Clarence. Once word got out that Edward had died, his half sister, Mary Tudor, began her plan to negate her brother's last will and testament and reclaim the throne. It was declared in the Parliament that Edward's last order as King was invalid. The Privy Council of Britain then switched their allegiances from Jane to that of Mary. Jane and Guilford were pronounced traitors and Jane declared a usurper of the throne, even though it was handed to her by the King. After only nine days in power, Jane and Guilford were arrested and locked in the Tower to await their trials. As expected, she and her husband were found guilty and sentenced to die.

However, the Imperial Ambassador reported to Charles V, the Holy Roman Emperor, that she was to be spared. It was a Protestant uprising that sealed Jane and Guilford's fates. Even though they were to be spared, the new Queen of England, Mary Tudor, was pressured into executing the young Royals to dispel any murmurings of any further rebellions. On February 12, 1554, both Jane and Guilford were beheaded, he in the public area of Tower Hill, and she in private on the Tower Green, a courtesy extended to her by the new Queen.

Nowadays, it is said that Lord Guilford Dudley's spirit appears in the Beauchamp Tower of the Tower of London, the tower in which he awaited his execution. He is often seen with soft tears running down his pallid cheek and the area in which he walks is said to be rife with poltergeist-like activity.

His bride, Lady Jane Grey, is said to wander the halls of the Salt Tower, with her most memorable appearance occurring on February 12, 1957. A guard of the tower reported seeing the figure of a sad, lonely young woman on one of the battlements above him as he patrolled the area. A second guard also caught sight of her spirit and both were seized with a heavy feeling of sadness.

Ironically, it was the 403rd anniversary of her execution.

The Princes of the Tower

Remember Henry VI, the mad king? And Henry's son Edward IV, who was killed in the Battle of Tewkesberry? When Henry VI died suddenly in May of 1483, followed by the death of his eldest son Edward IV, it was his 12-year-old son who was slated to succeed him as King Edward V. His 9-year-old brother, Richard, would follow his brother onto the throne should Edward not be able to fulfill his duties. But before he could be crowned, Parliament decreed that Edward and Richard, the two young princes, were illegitimate and thus ineligible for the crown. Their uncle, murderer of their father, assumed the throne as Richard III.

The princes were then placed in the Bloody Tower under the pretenses that they were to prepare for Edward's coronation, as this was the tradition for monarchs on the eves of their coronation. They were a familiar sight to the Beefeaters, or guards, of the Tower, playing happily on the Tower grounds. But in June of 1483, the boys vanished, never to be seen again. Rumor held that it was their uncle, the ambitious and villainous Richard III, who had them killed and buried somewhere on the grounds. In 1674, their tiny skeletons were discovered buried underneath a staircase in the famed White Tower. A Royal burial in Westminster Abbey followed as the two princes were laid to rest amongst their family.

Today, tourist and employee alike have seen the terror-stricken spirits of the two boys, dressed in their night clothes, clutching each other tightly in the rooms where they supposedly met their demise. Those who have encountered the spirits of Edward and Richard have reached out to console the terrified youngsters but are always rebuffed as they fearfully back away and disappear from view.

The Ghost of Anne Boelyln

Certainly the most famous King the British throne ever knew was King Henry VIII, whose preoccupation with the crumbling of the Roman Catholic Church's hold over the throne of England was fairly well known. Henry abhorred the idea of having to answer to the Church, and one of his first acts as King was to eradicate the influence of the Church over matters dealing with the throne of England. He did this by divorcing his first wife, Catherine of Aragon, which led to England's break with Rome and the starting of his own church, the Church of England. It can also be said that he wanted no hindrances to his rather fickle taste in women, which might be partly correct, but it was his wish to reign supreme and not have to answer to a Bishop, Cardinal, or Pope.

His impetus for divorcing Catherine Of Aragon? His desire to wed, then bed, Anne Boelyn, sister of one of his former mistresses. Anne begot a daughter to Henry, Elizabeth, but her next three pregnancies resulted in miscarriages. While Henry dearly loved his daughter, he could not bear to be without a male heir. It almost seemed like a gift that rumors of Anne's infidelity with her own brother, as well as accusations of treason had reached Henry's ears. She was tried and found guilty on all counts. At her public execution on the Tower Square, Anne chose to kneel upright, as was the custom for French executions. Her executioner, a skilled Frenchman named Jean Rombaud, was so shaken with the task that he found it difficult to proceed. Her last words were recorded as: "To Jesus Christ I commend my soul; Lord Jesus receive my soul."

Following the execution, Henry blew off a proper funeral for his wife, going so far as to leave her body on the scaffold for some time until a Tower workman had come across an old arrow chest that he used to store her body and head. Anne, once loved and revered Queen of England, was buried in an unmarked grave in the Chapel of St. Peter ad. Vincula. It wasn't until the renovations ordered by Queen Victoria in 1888 that her body was re-discovered and memorialized as Henry should have done 352 years before.

Perhaps the most famous spirit of the Tower of London, Anne has been seen on several occasions since her untimely execution. Her restless ghost walks the floors of the chapel of St. Peter ad Vincula, as well as The White Tower, the King's House, and the Tower Square, where she took her last breaths. Clad in her familiar black dress, the same one she is said to have been executed in, Anne walks mournfully through the night, oftentimes as a headless ghost carrying her head beneath her arm.

In 1864, a Beefeater on duty at the Tower encountered the headless ghost of Anne Boelyn. Stunned, he cautiously challenged her with his bayonet, but passed out cold when the blade passed straight through her, as if she were smoke. Facing a court marital for either sleeping or drinking on duty, he was saved by his fellow guards when they reported that his sighting of Anne's ghost was a common occurrence. Apparently, this was the guard's first encounter with the former Queen, but not likely to be his last.

Arthur Crick's Encounter

The account of Mr. Arthur Crick takes place in one of the walkways of The White Tower. The White Tower is considered to be one of the more haunted sections of the Tower of London, with reports of a Lady In White walking the halls and a dense, heavy feeling in Henry VIII's armory. Additionally, poltergeist activity has also been reported in the same armory, with one former guard reporting a physical attack that left red bruises on his neck.

That being said, there is no real idea where this story came from, nor are there any suggestions as to whose spirit spoke to Mr. Crick. I don't disbelieve the story in the least and Mr. Crick's reaction is priceless. Read on…

Arthur Crick was a Beefeater at the Tower of London whose duties included a night patrol in the White Tower. One night while on his rounds, Mr. Crick sat on a nearby ledge and took off his right shoe. As he massaged his aching foot, a voice from behind him whispered, "There's only you and I here," to which Arthur replied, "Just let me get this bloody shoe on and there'll only be you!"

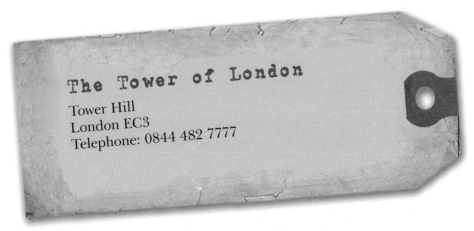

The Tower of London

Tower Hill
London EC3
Telephone: 0844 482 7777

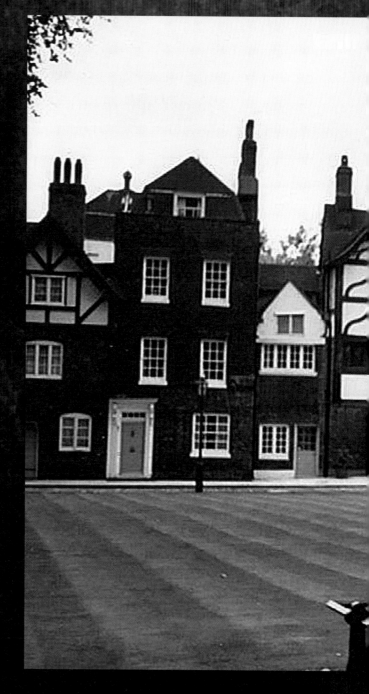

PHOTO 55 - TOWER OF LONDON PRIVATE EXECUTION
The Tudor's Home at the Tower of London. Near here are the private execution grounds where
subjects from Sir Walter Raleigh to Anne Boelyn breathed their last. *Photo courtesy of Linda*

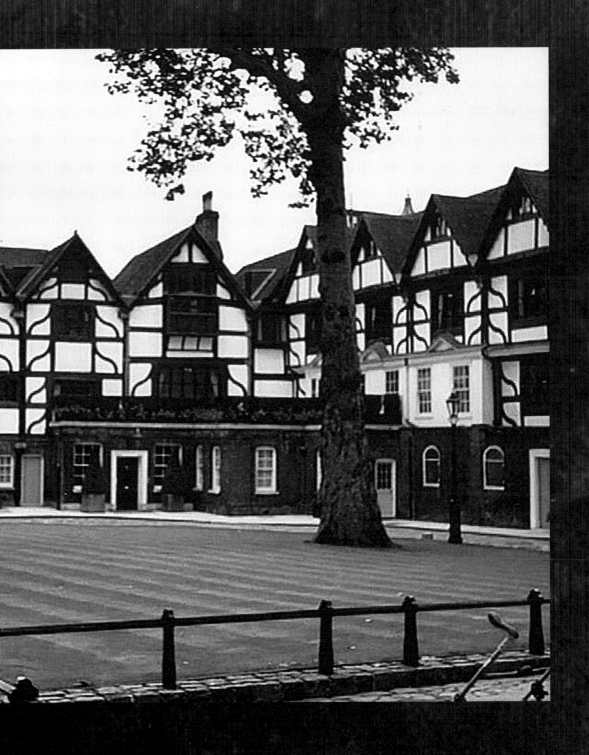

29.

AUSCHWITZ
Oswiecim, Poland
1941-1945

"The world is a dangerous place. Not because of the people who are evil, but because of the people who don't do anything about it."

~Albert Einstein

Though they are plentiful, the birds don't sing. Silence creeps throughout the empty barracks and buildings of Auschwitz I. An overwhelming sense of despondency and veneration washes over you as you step through the gates that once read "Arbeit Macht Frei (Work Will Make You Free)."

In Auschwitz II, only a few miles away in Birkenau, once you get past the imposing darkness of the train station, one finds nothing more than the bombed-out remains of several barracks, gas chambers, and incinerators.

For a long time, I debated whether or not I should include a chapter on the most infamous Nazi prison camp in history. As a paranormal investigator, it is an unwritten rule that concentration camps and places of general reverence and magnitude such as the World Trade Center or the Oklahoma City Federal Building were off limits to investigations and the like. Yet, as a writer and researcher, I find it is my duty to tell what I know, to pass on the knowledge I have thus far collected. Only one paranormal investigation has ever been performed at the Nazi concentration camps and it is doubtful one will ever be performed again, yet it is impossible to dismiss the feelings of wretchedness and sorrow that has drifted over this place of death and horror; it is a sadness that you take with you when you leave.

Of all of the haunted places in this book, this is perhaps the most haunted. Haunted by spirits, yes, but haunted by grief, horror, loss, regret, and fear as well. Of all of the Nazi-controlled concentration camps that dotted the East European landscapes of Poland and Czechoslovakia, it is the name Auschwitz that connects people with the atrocities committed against the Jews of Europe. To the Jewish people, Dachau, Bergen-Belsen, and other concentration camps held fear and mystery, as well as a fleeting hope that life could and would go on. But when the name Auschwitz passed their lips, they knew something else was going to happen. To see or hear about Auschwitz meant death, despair, and hopelessness. And they were right.

Auschwitz I originally began life as an old army barracks in Poland, built for Nazi soldiers stationed in Poland during the early days of World War II. But as their reign broadened and their hold on Europe tightened, the barracks were abandoned by the military as a base and quickly remodeled into efficient and lethal death camps for the millions of Jews being taken into custody as a part of Hitler's "Final Solution."

Construction on Auschwitz II began in 1941 as a way to alleviate the overcrowding at Auschwitz I. But there was a difference. According to Auschwitz commandant Rudolph Hoss, he had received orders from Heinrich Himmler, Hitler's second in command, that Auschwitz II was to be designed and built specifically for the quick and efficient extermination of the Jewish people. Hoss did not let Himmler down. Some shower rooms were retrofitted with pipes capable of delivering poisonous nerve gas called Xyclon B, and massive crematories were built to help dispose of the bodies of the dead. The camp was built around existing railroads to make the delivery of Jews and much needed supplies easier, and the remote isolation of the Polish countryside assured that the average trespasser or curious civilian would not be a problem. It was a place where, literally, no one would be able to hear you scream.

When the death camp began to receive its first inmates in 1941, Nazi officers segregated Jews based on their health, sex, and age. Sick and elderly Jews, as well as most children and their mothers normally were sent directly to the gas-equipped showers or the crematories where they could be executed and disposed of. Younger, healthier Jewish men were put to work in the camp, usually disposing of the bodies of their loved ones. Children who were selected to live were given their own barracks, as were the women.

If you were a set of Jewish twins, you would most likely receive a visit from Dr. Josef Mengele, the so-called "Angel Of Death," a German physician obsessed with human experimentation, especially regarding twins. When his experiments with the children had concluded, he had no trouble putting them out of their misery and exporting their skeletons to German medical schools. Mengele's twisted curiosities were met with fervor from the SS, who generously supplied him what he needed; his exploits, after all, were all to benefit the Nazi regime and the betterment of the Aryan race. His experiments ranged from what the effects of prolonged cold, poisons, and malaria had upon the body to the macabre surgeries and amputations of body parts. Mengele tried to create conjoined twins by sewing their hands and heads together. He had even injected experimental solutions into his subjects eyes in an effort to possibly change the eye color from brown to blue. Not one of his experiments yielded anything but death. Over 700 children died at Mengele's hands and he once personally ordered the deaths of close to 7,500 women infected with head lice, only because he felt it was easier than trying to treat an epidemic.

One of the more malicious guards on duty at Auschwitz II was Irma Grese, a stunning 22-year-old woman with a mean streak in her that ran to the bone. She delighted in turning her two vicious German Shepherds on the Jewish women for whom she was in charge, and gladly took part in arbitrary beatings and random shootings. Grese was quite promiscuous, not only with her SS superiors and fellow guards, but she also ordered Jewish prisoners to engage in sexual acts for her amusement. At only 22 years of age, she was already the second highest ranking female officer at Auschwitz II, having made marked impressions upon her supervisors while stationed at Ravensbruck and Bergen-Belsen concentration camps. Grese was put in charge of Crematory #3, selecting which Jews would be sent to die in the gas chambers and which would be spared. She may have been personally responsible for close to a million deaths during her time at Auschwitz II.

After four and a half years of torture, murder, and horror, Auschwitz II was liberated by Russia's Soviet Army as they made their way across Europe, pushing the Nazis back and spearheading the defeat of the Third Reich's plans for a Nazi dominated Europe. By the time World War II ended, over six million Jews had been murdered and disposed of in mass graves or in crematories such as the ones found in Auschwitz. As the War came to a close, Commandant Hoss, in an effort to cover up the Nazi's brutal activities, ordered the destruction of crematories and barracks before as many as 60,000 Jews were evacuated to Germany on a March of Death that claimed the lives of 15,000 en route.

Seven thousand remained behind at Auschwitz II, liberated by the Russian Army in 1945. They were the ones the Nazis had deemed too frail and sick to make the Death March back to Germany. They were the ones the Nazis had predicted would die sooner than later, yet they were the first ones liberated.

A year later, Commandant Hoss and Irma Grese, among others, were captured by Allied Forces and taken to Nuremburg, Germany to stand trial. Hoss estimated that while at Auschwitz II, he and his soldiers had taken the lives of close to 2,500,000 Jews. Both were quickly convicted and hanged for their part in Hitler's massive plan for the genocide of the Jewish peoples of Europe. Mengele, meanwhile, escaped and fled to Argentina, where he lived out the rest of his life.

Grese's death propelled her to icon status in Germany, as many believed that she had been a scapegoat for more corrupt SS officers who eluded capture by the Russians and the Allied Forces. Whether this is true or not is obviously up for debate, but the cult of those believing in Irma Grese's "innocence" was beginning to grow.

The Ghost of Irma Grese

A lot has been said about the possibility that SS auxiliary guard Irma Grese's spirit still walks the hallowed ground of Auschwitz II. While smidgens of truth may lie inside fictitious details, it is unrealistic to pick apart which are truths and which are lies. Here is the general story and I'll let you decide.

In 1947, Auschwitz II was officially opened to the public as a museum dedicated to the Holocaust of Jews in Eastern Europe. And at almost the same time the museum opened, the experiences began, most notably with the hauntings of Crematory #3 with appearances of the radiant, yet brutal Irma Grese inside the horrific building that helped to take the lives of 2.5 million Jews.

Rumors and gossip about Irma's ghost started early on following her death in 1945. On January 12, 1948, night watchman Harak Visen reported that he once saw Irma Grese's ghost in Crematory #3 while doing his rounds. A suspicious photograph turned up showing the misty figure of a woman walking between two crematory ovens. Sightings and experiences became so prevalent that the Russian caretakers in charge of keeping Auschwitz up decided to seal off Crematory #3 in 1948. It remained sealed until 1992 when a Jewish parapsychologist named Heim Lansky led a crew on an investigation of the Crematory. It is rumored that they did not last through the night and the investigation was aborted early. Crematory #3 was resealed, then finally destroyed. Reports of Irma's ghost abruptly ceased.

But did it really happen that way?

It is no secret that much of Auschwitz II was destroyed by the Nazis as they fled in a vain attempt to cover up what they had done. If every gas chamber and crematory was already destroyed, how could the Russians in charge of Auschwitz lock up anything? Pictures of the site show a bombed-out Crematory #3, with no ovens, or walls at all. Only rubble. That alone invalidates the story as a pure truth. There may have been elements of truth once before, but they have since become watered down, oversimplified, and falsified to the point of farce.

The Personal Experiences

When sudden death or prolonged terror occur, it can create deep welts in the spaces where they happened. It is impossible to not feel thousands of invisible faces watching you as you step through the gates of Auschwitz, nor is it possible to quell the blanket-like feeling of melancholy that only tightens the longer you stay. Could there be a residual feeling of terror, sadness, and confusion plaguing Auschwitz I and II?

People have reported feeling claustrophobic, even in large, open spaces, with hundreds of invisible eyes watching them. These tourists and sightseers get the overwhelming feeling that they are experiencing what the Jews of 1940-1945 must have felt while disembarking the trains inside the death camp. It begins as they step past the gates and alleviates only when they exit.

Multiple cold spots have been reported in the fields, followed by static charges that rifle through the body of those fortunate enough to experience it. To paranormal investigators, it is this static feeling of electromagnetic energy that signifies the presence of a spirit. Photographs taken in the remaining crematories, barracks, and shower rooms of Auschwitz have revealed mist-like apparitions, shadows, and orbs, as well as unexplained light anomalies that seem to have no source.

In Block 10, which served as Josef Mengele's medical building, there have been rumors of hearing the voices of children, small voices speaking in Hungarian, Russian, and Polish dialects and languages.

As people enter the children's barracks and gas chambers of Auschwitz I, they have felt warm, unseen hands reach out and clasp their own. What is felt is anything but horrific or terrifying. It is an almost soothing and welcome touch from the past, a soft grab of desperate hands reaching out to those who still live, an effort to embrace the life they once knew or perhaps comfort those who still mourn.

Perhaps the most touching, yet alternately chilling, experience has to be when a young woman felt a slight tugging on her clothes and a small, unseen voice whispered to her. The woman, a Hungarian, immediately recognized her native language, though she could not decipher all the words. What words she did hear made her break down into sobs: "Kérem hagyjuk," it had said. "Please, leave."

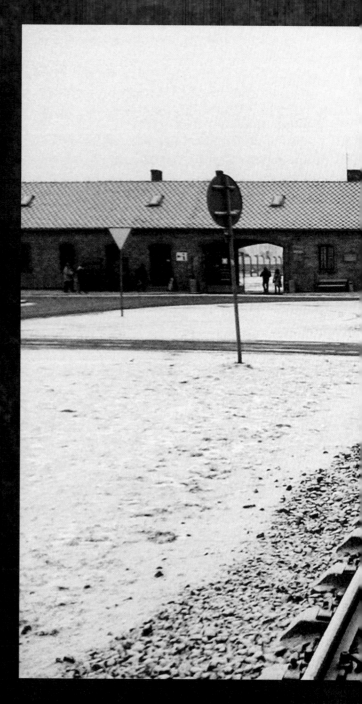

PHOTO 22-AUSCHWITZ II TRAIN
Photo courtesy of Julian Alexe.

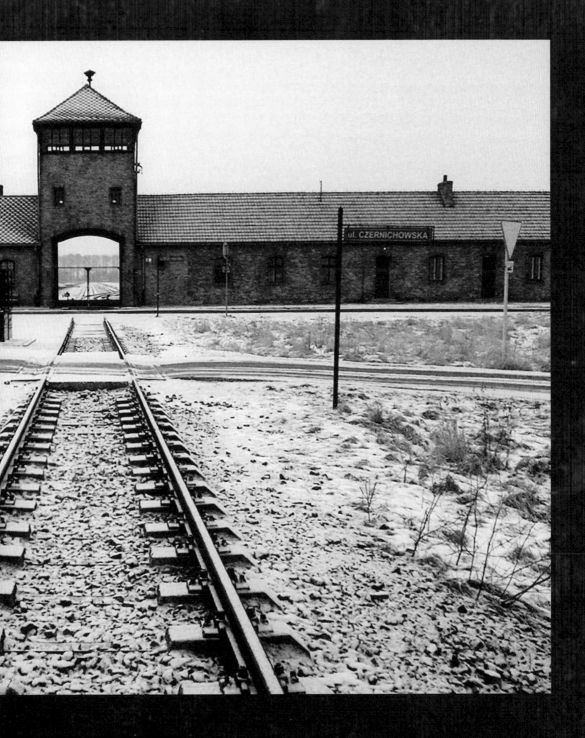

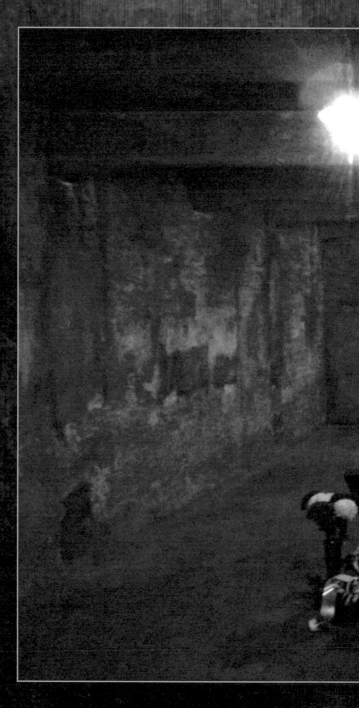

PHOTO 25 - AUSCHWITZ I GAS CHAMBER
One of the gas chambers at Auschwitz I. *Photo courtesy of Julian Alexe.*

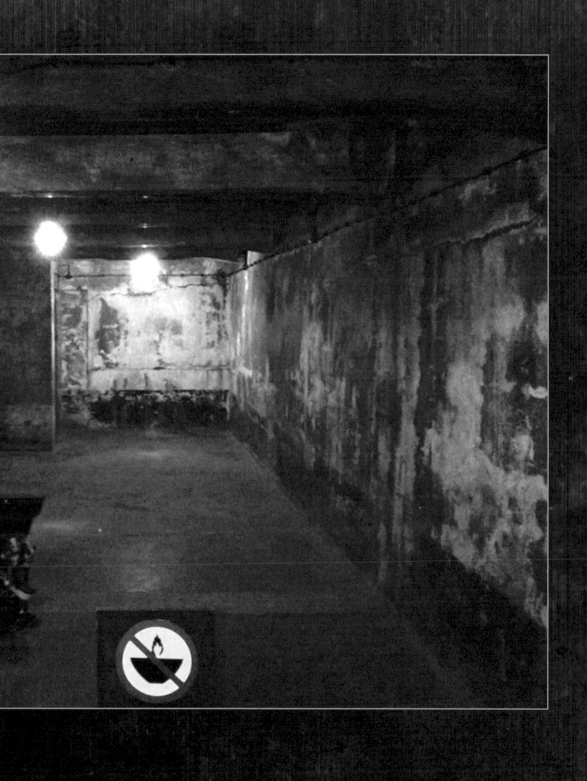

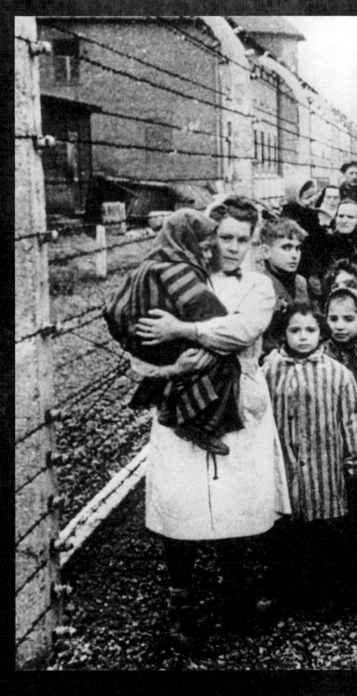

PHOTO 30 - AUSCHWITZ II CHILDREN

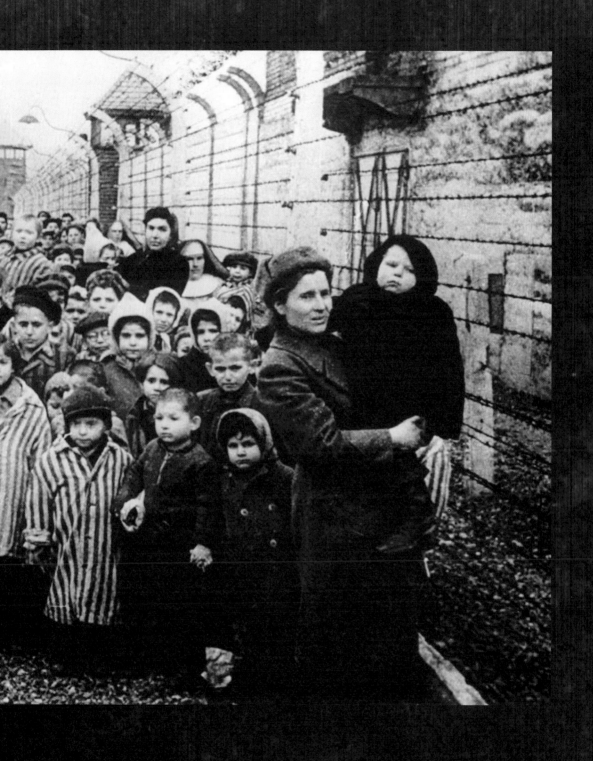

Appendix One
SELECTED RESOURCES

WEST VIRGINIA STATE PENITENTIARY

Associated Press. "Hostage Forced To Watch Killing During Prison Riot, Guards Say." *The Palm Beach Post.* Palm Beach, FL. January 6, 1986

Associated Press. "Hostages Recall Prison Seizure Brutality." The Vindicator. Youngstown, OH. January 6, 1986

Ghost Adventures (TV) Episode #3. "Moundsville State Penitentiary." 2008. The Travel Channel

Ghost Stories (TV) Episode #1.04. "Moundsville Prison." The Travel Channel. October 23, 2009

Montaldo, Charles. "Haunting Ghost Stories of West Virginia Penitentiary: Plagued With Residual Haunting?" http://crime.about.com/od/prison/a/moundsvills.htm

Morgan, Sue (UPI). "Snyder Trial Up in the Air." *Point Pleasant Register.* Point Pleasant, WV. March 16, 1989

Most Haunted Places in America. "Moundsville State Penitentiary." http://www.ghosteyes.com/haunmoundsville-state-penitentiary

Visions Magazine. "Interview With Psychic Nancy Meyers." http://www.youtube.com/watch?v=GZkFzSkqxbw

West Virginia State Penitentiary Official Website. http://www.wvpentours.com/

WAVERLY HILLS SANATORIUM

Belanger, Jeff. "Waverly Hills Sanatorium." *The World's Most Haunted Places, Revised Edition.* New Page Books. Pompton Plains, NJ. 2011

Brown, Alan. *Haunted Kentucky: Ghosts & Strange Phenomena Of The Blue Grass State.* Stackpole Books. Mechanicsburg, PA. 2009

Waverly Hills Sanatorium Official Website. www.therealwaverlyhills.com

Bryan, Bobette. "Waverly Hills Sanitarium: The Haunted Hospital." http://www.underworld-tales.com/waverly.htm

Ghost Adventures (TV) Episode #30. "Waverly Hills Sanatorium." 2010.

Ghost Hunters (TV) Episode #214. "Waverly Hills." March 29, 2006

Ghost-Story.co.uk. "Waverly Hills Sanatorium." www.ghost-story.co.uk/stories/waverlyhill-sroom502.html

Ray, Becky. "Waverly Hills Sanatorium." Ghost-Investigators.com. http://www.ghost-nves-tigators.com/Stories/view_story.php?story_num=27

Smith, Christian. "Armaments of Health." Saskatoon Star-Phoenix, 1938. http://www.lung.ca/tb/tbhistory/treatment/heliotherapy.html

Taylor, Troy. *America's Most Haunted Places.* "Waverly Hills Sanatorium." http://www.prairieg-hosts.com/waverly_tb.html

ANDERSONVILLE PRISON

Belanger, Jeff. *Ghosts of War: Restless Spirits of Soldiers, Spies, and Saboteurs.* New Page Books. Pompton Plains, NJ. 2006.

GhostWriter. "Andersonville Prison Still Haunts." http://www.ghosteyes.com/anderson-ville-prison-haunts

HauntedPlacesToGo.com "The Hauntings of the Andersonville Prison in Andersonville, Georgia." www.haunted-places-to-go.com/andersonville-prison.html

Hector, Erin. "The Ghosts of Andersonville." www.associatedcontent.com/article/2402634/the_ghosts_of_Andersonville.html

Hometown Tales (VIDEO) "The Horrors of Andersonville." http://www.youtube.com/watch?v=d6w0S0KmHws

Stefko, Jill. "Haunted Andersonville Prison." www.suite101.com/content/haunted-anderson-ville-prison-a110370

ANCORA PSYCHIATRIC HOSPITAL VILLAGE

Haunted Sites in New Jersey. home.comcast.net/~parainvestigator/NJ/NewJersey.html

The LostInJersey Blog. "The Abandoned Patient Houses of Ancora Psychiatric." http://lostinjersey.wordpress.com/2009/03/18/the-abandoned-patient-houses-of-ancora-psychi-atric/

GREYSTONE PARK PSYCHIATRIC HOSPITAL

Garner, Craig B. "Lost Hospital: Greystone Park Psychiatric Hospital." January 19, 2011. http://hospitalstay.com/2011/01/lost-hospital-greystone-park-psychiatric-hospital-morris-town-new-jersey/

KirkbrideBuildings.com. "Greystone Park." http://www.kirkbridebuildings.com/buildings/greystonepark/

UrbanExploration.com. "New Jersey State Hospital For The Insane." http://www.forbidden-places.net/urban-exploration-New-Jersey-State-Hospital-for-the-insane

ESSEX COUNTY HOSPITAL

Allison, Andrea. "Ghost Stories: Essex County Hospital Center." http://paranormalstories.blogspot.com/2009/04/essex-county-mental-hospital.html. April 29, 2009

ROLLING HILLS ASYLUM

Allison, Andrea. "Rolling Hills." http://paranormalstories.blogspot.com/2007/06/rolling-hills.html

Conklin, Susan L. "History of The Genesee County Poorhouse." http://rollinghillsasylum.com/

Ghost Adventures (TV) Episode #28. "Rolling Hills Asylum." September 24, 2010.

Ghost Hunters (TV) Episode #209. "Dave Tango & Rolling Hills."

Ghost Adventures. "Rolling Hills' Haunting History." The Travel Channel

Gypsy1Witch. "The Legend Of Rolling Hills Asylum" www.gypsy1with.hubpages.com/hub/The-Legend-Of-Rolling-Hills-Asylum-Bethany-NY

Real Haunted Places in America: Rolling Hills Asylum. http://www.haunted-places-to-go.com/rolling-hills-asylum.html

www.paranormal.about.com/od/hauntedplaces/ig/World-s-Most-Haunted-Place/Rolling-Hills-Asylum.htm

DANVERS STATE HOSPITAL

AsylumProjects.org. "Danvers State Hospital." www.asylumprojects.org/index.php?title=Danvers_State_Hospital

Puffer, Michael. "The Lore—and lure—of Danvers Hospital." *Danvers Herald.* www.haunted-salem.com/news/oct03-dh-danversstate.html. October 29, 2003

EASTERN STATE PENITENTIARY

Chirico, Dina A., and Joan Upton Hall, editor. "An Experiment In: Solitude Eastern State Penitentiary." *Ghostly Tales From America's Jails.* Atriad Press. Dallas, TX. 2006

Eastern State Penitentiary Official Website. www.easternstate.org

Ghost Adventures (TV) Episode #14. "Eastern State Penitentiary." July 10, 2009

Ghost Hunters (TV) Episode #105. "Eastern State Penitentiary." November 3, 2004

Taylor, Troy. PrairieGhosts.com "History & Hauntings of Eastern State Penitentiary." http://www.prairieghosts.com/eastern.html

TheCabinet.com. Dark Destinations. "Eastern State Penitentiary." www.thecabinet.com/darkdestinations

Wagner, Stephen. *World's Most Haunted Places.* "Eastern StatePenitentiary." www.paranormal.about.com/od/hauntedplaces/ig/World-s-Most-Haunted-Place/Eastern-State-Penitentiary.htm

PRESTON CASTLE

Allison, Andrea. "Preston School of Industry." http://paranormalstories.blogspot.com/2009/06/preston-castle.html. 2009

Budd, Deena. "Paranormal Site: Preston Castle." www.bellaonline.com/articles/art65507.asp

Ghost Adventures (TV) Episode #9. "Preston Castle." June 5, 2009

Ghost Hunters (TV) Episode #606. "Haunted Reform School." April 7, 2010

GhostEyes.com. "Haunted Preston Castle." www.ghosteyes.com/haunted-preston-castle-ione-california

Haunted Places To Go. "The Mysteries of The Preston Castle in Ione, CA." http://www.haunted-places-to-go.com/haunted-castle-1.html

Preston Castle Foundation. "History." http://www.prestoncastle.com/tours.html.

Rubio, J'Aime. "Who Was Anna Corbin?" http://dreamingcasuallypoetry.blogspot.com/2011/06/who-was-anna-corbin.html. June 9, 2011.

Unknown. "Preston Castle Investigation." http://www.packrat-pro.com/ghost/prestoncastle.htm

ASHMORE ESTATES

Ashmore Estates Official Website. www.ashmoreestates.net/home.html

Clark, Bonnie. "Coles County Poor Farm: Local Resident Recalls Memories of Living There

During her Childhood." *Journal Gazette & Times Courier*

Ghost Adventures (TV) Episode #54. "Ashmore Estates." September 23, 2011

http://jg-tc.com/lifestyles/article_7c7e2893-2703-5fae-89a2-07e93a4a7965.html. October 19, 2009

BARTONVILLE STATE HOSPITAL

Clifton-Pennell, Penny. "Central Illinois Insane Asylum." February 23, 2008. http://www.associatedcontent.com/article/619011/central_illinois_insaneasylum_haunted.html?cat=16

Taylor, Troy. "The Bartonville Insane Asylum." c. 2000. http://www.prairieghosts.com/barton.html

WYOMING FRONTIER PRISON

Allison, Andrea. "Wyoming Frontier Prison." http://paranormalstories.blogspot.com/2009/09/wyoming-frontier-prison.html. September 18, 2009

HauntedHouses.com. "Wyoming Frontier Prison." http://www.hauntedhouses.com/states/wy/frontier-prison.cfm

HauntedPlacesToGo.com. "The Haunted Frontier Prison In Rawlings, Wyoming." http://www.haunted-places-to-go.com/haunted-prison-3.html

Wyoming Frontier Prison Official Website. http://wyomingfrontierprison.org/

CENTRAL STATE MENTAL INSTITUTION

Ancestry.com. "History of Central State Hospital aka Central State Hospital For The Insane." http://www.rootsweb.ancestry.com/~asylums/central_in/index.html

Associated Press. "Hospital Death is Being Investigated." *The Madison Courier.* March 24, 1992

Eblin, Jennifer. "The Ghosts of Central State Hospital in Indianapolis." Yahoo! Network contributor. http://www.associatedcontent.com/article/415949/the_ghosts_of_central_state_hospital.html

Hall, Dan T. (Director/Writer) *Central State: Asylum For The Insane.* 2006. Vizmo Films

Hancock, Shane. *Doing Indy: Central State Mental Hospital Part I* (VIDEO) http://www.youtube.com/user/film1999#p/a/u/2/edAQTq-3SUQg

Hancock, Shane. *Doing Indy: Central State Mental Hospital Part II* VIDEO) http://www.youtube.com/user/film1999#p/a/u/0/Za6d799eueI

HauntedHouses.com. "Central State Hospital." www.hauntedhouses.com/states/in/indiana_central_state_hospital.cfm

Ksander, Yael. "Central State Hospital." *Indiana Public Media.* http://indianapublicmedia.org/momentofindianahistory/central-state-hospital/

Merriman, Mark. "When Darkness Comes To Central State." *Haunted Indiana 3.* http://www.prairieghosts.com/central_state.html

Sankowsky, Lorri and Keri Young. *Ghost Hunters Guide To Indianapolis.* Pelican Publications. Gretna, Louisiana. 2008

OHIO STATE REFORMATORY

Belanger, Jeff. "Mansfield Reformatory." *The World's Most Haunted Places*, Revised Edition. New Page Books. Pompton Plains, NJ. 2011

DeadOhio.com. "Mansfield Reformatory." http://www.deadohio.com/mansfieldreformatory.htm

Ghost Adventures (TV) Episode #20. "Ohio State Reformatory." 2009

Ghosts of Ohio. "Ohio State Reformatory." http://www.ghostsofohio.org/lore/ohio_lore_33.html

Haunted-Houses.com. "Ohio State Reformatory."http://www.hauntedhouses.com/states/oh/ohio_state_pen.cfm

Lore, David. "Inside the Pen." *The Columbus Dispatch.* http://www.mrps.org/pages/inside-the-pen

Ohio State Reformatory Official Website. www.mrps.org

Olson, Lynne. "Ohio State Reformatory." Mediumlynneolson.wordpress.com http://mediumlynneolson.wordpress.com/2010/09/11/ohio-reformatory/

Santore, Beth. "Ohio State Reformatory." GraveAddiction.com.http://www.graveaddiction.com/osr.html

United Press. "Brutal Slaying of Three Starts Biggest Manhunt Since Dillinger's Day." *The Pittsburgh Press.* Pittsburgh, PA. July 22, 1948

ALCATRAZ FEDERAL PENITENTIARY

Esslinger, Michael. *Alcatraz: A Definitive History Of The Penitentiary Years.* Ocean View Publishing. Sarasota, FL. July 24, 2011

Ghost Hunters (TV) Episode #601. "Alcatraz." March 3, 2010

Montaldo, Charles. "Is Al Capone Still Wandering the Corridors of Alcatraz?" www.crime.about.com/od/prison/a/alcatrazghosts.htm

Mysteries of the Unexplained (TV). "Psychic Peter James Visits Alcatraz." http://www.youtube.com/watch?v=DnYPAGwSmNk

Taylor, Troy. Compiled by Joanne Austin. "Ghosts of Alcatraz." *Weird Hauntings*. Sterling Publishing. New York, NY. 2006

Taylor, Troy. "Doing Time for Eternity on The Rock: The Hauntings of Alcatraz." http://www.prairieghosts.com/gpalcatraz.html

YourGhostStories.com. "The Hauntings of Alcatraz." http://www.yourghoststories.com/famous-ghost-stories/alcatraz-hauntings.php

YORKTOWN MEMORIAL HOSPITAL

Ghost Adventures (TV) Episode #47. "Yorktown Memorial." March 18, 2011

Haunted Places in Texas. "Yorktown Memorial Hospital." http://www.haunted-places-to-go.com/haunted-places-in-texas-1.html

Olson, Lynne. "Ghost Adventures: Yorktown Memorial Hospital." www.mediumlynneolson.wordpress.com

Rush, Russell. "Haunted Tour." http://www.mix961.com/pages/hauntedtour/yorktown.html

Victoria Advocate. "A Night At Yorktown Hospital." http://www.victoriaadvocate.com/news/2011/apr/02/kb_paranormal_040311_134828/?entertainment&local-entertainment

TRANS-ALLEGHENY LUNATIC ASYLUM

Darling, J. *Haunted Places.* "Trans-Allegheny Lunatic Asylum in Weston, West Virginia." www.associatedcontent.com/article/2497087/haunted_place_the_transallegheny_lunatic.html?cat=16

Ghost Adventures (TV) Episode #17. "The Trans-Allegheny Lunatic Asylum." The Travel Channel. 2009

Ghost Hunters (TV) Episode #409. "Haunted Asylum." SyFy Channel. April 30, 2008

Ghost Stories. (TV) Episode 1.01. "Trans-Allegheny." The Travel Channel. October 16, 2009

GhostEyes.com. Most Haunted Places in America. "Trans-Allegheny Lunatic Asylum." ghosteyes.com/transallegheny-lunatic-asylum-hauntings

GypsyWitch1. "The Story of Trans-Allegheny Lunatic Asylum." http://hubpages.com/hub/The-Story-of-Tran-Allegheny-Lunatic-Asylum

HubPages.com. "Trans-Allegheny Lunatic Asylum Facts and Fiction." http://hubpages.com/hub/Trans-Allegheny-Lunatic-Asylum-Facts-and-Fiction

Logisti. "GH: Trans-Allegheny Lunatic Asylum." SkepticalViewer.com. www.skepticalviewer.com/2008/04/30/trans-allegheny-lunatic-asylum/

Muller, Rebecca. "Trans-Allegheny Lunatic Asylum." http://rebeccashott.com/#/trans-allegheny/4536950193

Trans-Allegheny Lunatic Asylum Official Website. http://www.trans-alleghenylunaticasylum.com/main/history.html

Wickline, John. "TAPS: Weston Hospital is Haunted." InterMountain.com. http://www.theintermountain.com/page/content.detail/id/506592.html

LINDA VISTA COMMUNITY HOSPITAL

Bucky. "The Haunting of Linda Vista Hospital." http://www.bloggingwv.com/the-hauntings-of-linda-vista-hospital/. July 10, 2007

Ghost Adventures (TV) Episode #23. "Linda Vista Hospital." December 11, 2009.

Ghost Stories (TV) Episode 2.12. "Dr. Edwards." The Travel Channel. October 22, 2010

OLD IDAHO STATE PENITENTIARY

Cuff, Marie & Julie Decker. Compiled by Joanne Austin. "The Old Idaho State Penitentiary." *Weird Hauntings*. Sterling Publishing Co. New York, NY. 2006

Ford, L.L. "Haunted History: The Old Idaho State Penitentiary."

Ghost Adventures (TV) Episode #8. "Old Idaho Penitentiary." December 5, 2008

Idaho State Historical Society. "The Old Idaho State Penitentiary." http://history.idaho.gov/old-idaho-penitentiary

NORWICH STATE HOSPITAL

Allison, Andrea. "Norwich State Hospital." http://paranormalstories.blogspot.com/2010/04/norwich-state-hospital.html. April 28, 2010

Bendici, Ray. "Norwich State Hospital, Preston." DamnedCT.com. http://www.damnedct.com/norwich-state-hospital-preston

Choiniere, Paul. "Former Norwich State Hospital Worker Preserves Memories." *Meridian Record-Journal.* January 23, 2007

GreatestUnsolvedMysteries.com. "Haunted Hospitals—Norwich State Hospital." http://www.greatest-unsolved-mysteries.com/Norwich-state-hospital.html

CLOVIS WOLFE MANOR

Clovis Wolfe Manor blog. http://kellyskrazynews.blogspot.com/2010/02/clovis-wolfe-manor-ghostly-sanitarium.html

Constantino, Mark and Debby. "Clovis Manor Investigation." Spirts-Speak.com www.spirits-speak.com/investigations_wolfe.html

Ghost Adventures (TV) Episode #26. "Clovis Wolfe Manor." January 8, 2010

Ghost Adventures Recap: Clovis Wolfe Manor. http://syfyghosthunters.blogspot.com/2010/01/ghost-adventures.html

Ghost Hunters (TV) Episode #425. "Recycled Souls." November 19, 2008

Martinez Paranormal. *The Haunted Wolfe Manor Hotel* (VIDEO). http://www.youtube.com/watch?v=Xl0Hv24iTvE

Most Haunted Places in America: Clovis Wolfe Manor. http://www.ghosteyes.com/clovis-wolfe-manor-hauntings

Ritchie, Ashley and Kyra Jenkins. "Mystery at the Mansion: Part 1" www.kmph.com/story/8682139/mystery-at-the-mansion-part-1?ClientType=Prinatable&redirected=true

BURLINGTON COUNTY PRISON

BecauseILive. "Haunted Places: Burlington County Prison." http://becauseilive.hubpages.com/hub/Haunted_Places_Burlington_County_Prison_Museum

Clough, Joel. *The Only True and Authentic Life and Confession of Joel Clough.* Published by Robert Desilver, Philadelphia. 1833. http://pds.lib.harvard.edu/pds/view/5809806

Ghost Stories (TV) Episode 2.11. "Joel Clough." The Travel Channel. October 22, 2010

Marsh, Roger. "The Short Life and Death of Joel Clough." Examiner.com. examiner.com/ufo-in-national/the-short-life-and-death-of-joel-clough. January 21, 2009

Philbrick, Kate. "The Haunted Burlington County Prison, Mount Holly." WeirdNJ.com http://www.weirdnj.com/index.php?option=com_content&task=view&id=18&Itemid=28

PENNHURST STATE SCHOOL

About Pennhurst State School And Hospital. http://preservepennhurst.org/default.aspx?pg=36

Ghost Adventures. "Pennhurst States Haunted History." http://www.travelchannel.com/TV_Shows/Ghost_Adventures

Ghost Adventures (TV) Episode #18. "Pennhurst State School." November 6, 2009

Ghost Hunters (TV) Episode #702. "Pennsylvania Asylum." March 2, 2011

Most Haunted Places in America: Pennhurst State Hopsital. http://www.ghosteyes.com/paranormal-activity-pennhurst-state-school

Preserve Pennhurst Official Website. www.preservepennhurst.org

Suffer The Little Children (Video) NBC10 Philadelphia. 1968.http://preservepennhurst.org/default.aspx?pg=26

LEAVENWORTH DISCIPLINARY BARRACKS

Brendel, Dale. "Is Fort Leavenworth Really Haunted? You Decide." Leavenworth Times.com. www.leavenworthtimes.com/features/x268458402/Q5-Local-hauntings-you-decide. October 19, 2011

Weiser, Kathy. "Fort Leavenworth." LegendsOfAmerica.com. http://www.legendsofamerica.com/ks-fortleavenworth.html. March, 2011

MADISON STATE HOSPITAL

Asylum Projects. "Madison State Hospital." http://www.asylumprojects.org/index.php?title=Madison_State_Hospital

Eblin, Jennifer. "A Haunted Tour of Madison, Indiana." http://www.associatedcontent.com/article/1046527/a_haunted_tour_of_madison_indiana.html?cat=8. September 28, 2008

INDIANA VETERANS HOME

StrangeUSA.com. "Indiana Veteran's Home (Pyle Building.)" http://www.strangeusa.com/Viewlocation.aspx?id=63881 FaceBook.com. www.facebook.com/pages/Indiana-Veterans-Home

OLD CHANGI HOSPITAL

http://real-ghosts-webs.blogspot.com/2011/01/most-haunted-place-in-singapore-old.html

http://remembersingapore.wordpress.com/old-changi-hospital/

http://spi.com.sg/haunted/haunted_changi/och.htm

POVEGLIA ISLAND

Awesome Mysteries You've Never Heard of. "Island of Madness." ww.slightlywarped.com/crapfactory/awesomemysteries/islandofmadness.htm

Belanger, Jeff. "Poveglia Island." *The World's Most Haunted Places*. Revised Edition. New Page Books. Pompton Plains, NJ. 2011

Ghost Adventures (TV) Episode #19. "Poveglia Island." November 13, 2009

Jfrater. "Poveglia: Island Of Terror." http://cog-itz.com/2010/03/22/poveglia-island-of-terror/

COVENANTERS PRISON & GREYFRIARS CEMETERY

Armstrong, Ruth. "Graverobbers Steal Skull in Tomb." http://edinburghnews.scotsman.com/edinburgh/Graverobbers-steal-skull-in-tomb.2440338.jp. July 2, 2003

Covenanter.org. "History of The Covenanters." http://www.covenanter.org.uk/Greyfriars/

Maclean, Diane. "The Tourist Terrorizing Mackenzie Poltergeist." www.heritage.scotsman.com/myths/The-touristterrorising-Mackenzie-poltergeist.2596627.jp. January 2005

Scottish Paranormal Investigations. "Greyfriars Kirkyard." www.scottishparanormalinvestigations.co.uk/investigations/greyfriars-kirkyard/

ABU GHRAIB PRISON

al-Muktar, Uthman. "Ghosts Of Abu Ghraib Still Haunt Local Sunnis." Institute of War and Peace. December 17, 2010

Goodwin, David. "Cries In The Dark: The Ghosts Of Abu Ghraib Prison." http://www.militaryghosts.com/prison.html

IPWR. December 22, 2010. http://www.isn.ethz.ch/isn/Current-Affairs/ISN-Insights/Detail?lng=en&id=125828&contextid734=125828&contextid735=125826&tabid=125826

THE TOWER OF LONDON

Belanger, Jeff. *The World's Most Haunted Places, Revised Edition.* New Page Books. Pompton Plains, NJ. 2011

EnglishMonarchs.co.uk. "Tower of London." http://www.englishmonarchs.co.uk/tower_london.htm

AUSCHWITZ-BIRKENAU CONCENTRATION CAMP

Branson-Trent, Gregory. "The Dead of Auschwitz-Birkenau Concentration Camp, Oswiecim, Poland." http://gregorybranson-trentsghosthuntersblog.blogspot.com/2010/10/dead-of-auschwitz-birkenau.html. October 24, 2010

Creager, Ellen. "Ghosts of Auschwitz Haunt Visitors." *Detroit Free Press*. http://www.post-gazette.com/pg/08222/900915-37.stm. August 9, 2008

EsotericOnline.com "The Ghost Files." Valerie, Paranormal Reporter. http://esotericonline.tripod.com/esotericonline_the_ghost_files.htm

Parizo, Chris. "The Hauntings of Auschwitz and Other Concentration Camps." *The Contrarian*. www.thecontrarianmedia.com/2009/10/the-hauntings-of-auschwitz-and-other-concentration-camps/

Appendix II
CONTRIBUTING PHOTOGRAPHERS

I absolutely love my photographers. Finding them was an integral part of writing this book; each of them had such a wholly original view of these majestic buildings. Their eyes found the intrinsic beauty within the decay and remained perfectly honest to the subject matter, a perspective that I had hoped to capture with my writing. Their view of these worlds inspired me to no end, and I thank each of them for allowing me to use their art for *Lost in the Darkness*. Please check out their Flickr Photostreams and enjoy their own unique view of the world around us. You'll be inspired as well.

Lori Mattas
Preston Castle
Owner, Mattas Media
www.mattasmedia.com

Lisa Katherine
Alcatraz
Flickr Photostream: www.flickr.com/photos/48225317@N08/

Mattie Parfitt
Preston Castle
Flickr Photostream: www.flickr.com/photos/38250858@N04/

Hannah Chervitz
Pennhurst State School
Flickr Photostream: www.flickr.com/photos/hannahlin/

Aimee Lindell
{beautiful}Lemons Photography
Norwich State Hospital
Flickr Photostream: www.flickr.com/photos/beautifullemons/

APPENDIX III
HOW TO SAVE THESE BUILDINGS

Most of these buildings are starting to crumble with time and the elements. Their historic value is known, but unappreciated. These buildings are a gateway to our past, as well as a cautionary reminder for our future. Preservation Societies are created by community members to salvage, renovate, and honor places that should be saved. They do a magnificent job of memorializing those who suffered there and try to keep alive the memory of those who called these places home. A few are listed below. Please take some time to look into the following Preservation Societies and help in any way you can.

PENNHURST STATE SCHOOL
www.preservepennhurst.com

WAVERLY HILLS SANATORIUM
www.therealwaverlyhills.com

WEST VIRGINIA STATE PENITENTIARY
www.wvpentours.com

OHIO STATE REFORMATORY
The Mansfield Reformatory Preservation Society
www.mrps.com

PRESTON CASTLE
The Preston Castle Foundation
www.prestoncastle.com

BURLINGTON COUNTY PRISON
www.prisonmuseum.net

CENTRAL STATE INSANE ASYLUM
Indiana Medical History Museum
Located on the grounds of Central State
www.imhm.org

GREYSTONE PARK PSYCHIATRIC HOSPITAL
www.preservegreystone.org

THE TRANS-ALLEGHENY LUNATIC ASYLUM
www.trans-alleghenylunaticasylum.com

ACKNOWLEDGMENTS

My fearless and wonderful editor, Dinah Roseberry.

The staff of Waverly Hills, West Virginia Penitentiary, Ohio State Reformatory, and the Trans-Allegheny Lunatic Asylum (especially my tour guide, Patrick).

My amazing photographers: Aimee Lindell, Lisa Katherine, Ryan Wirth, Brett Flick, Robert Schoneman, Lori Mattas, Sally Neate, Kevin Husta, Hannah Chervitz, Julian Alexe, and Mattie Parfitt.

Polly Gear, for allowing me to use her Shadow Man photograph.

My literary heroes Troy Taylor and Jeff Belanger, whose tireless work and research consistently proves invaluable, not only to me, but to everyone in the field.

And last, but not least, to you, the readers of my book who took the time to pick it up and support me in the culmination of a 30+ year dream to write and publish my own book. It's going to be a great ride, so stick with me and we'll see it through to the end together.

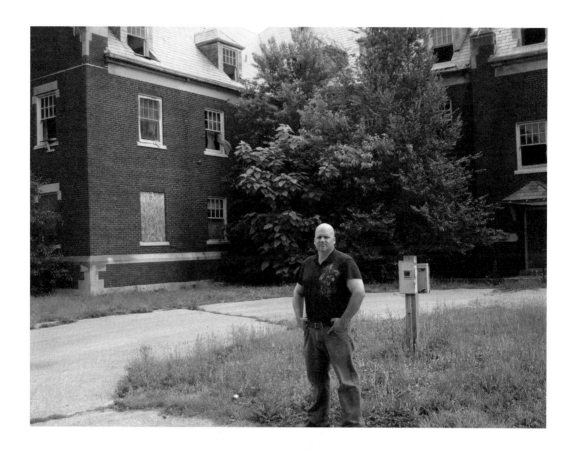

ABOUT THE AUTHOR

Benjamin S. Jeffries

Born in 1971 to theater-loving hippy intellectuals, Benjamin always held a fascination with the paranormal, a love that was solidified in 1982 when a photograph of him was taken that revealed an entity in the background that he named "John."

Since then, Benjamin has written stories, essays, and film scripts dealing with the dark heart of this reality and the reality beyond. He is the founder/lead investigator/psychic intuitive of the Wyandotte Paranormal Society, a ghost-hunting group based in the Lafayette-Dayton, Indiana area. He is also the author of *ACT III: A COLLECTION OF NOVELLAS*, the world's most horrendous attempt at writing serious fiction.

Benjamin lives with his beloved wife, Diane; their son, Brody; one lovable, loyal basset hound; one surly, but determined cat; three goldfish; two snails; and two very benign spirits who have yet to reveal their names, but enjoy his basement and upstairs closet very much.

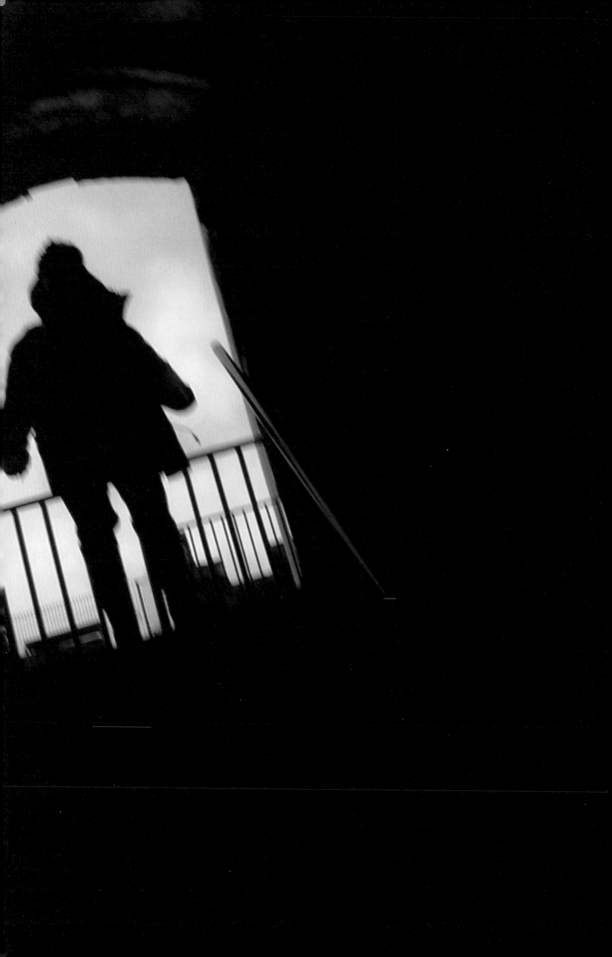